PHYLLIS SPEIGHT

Homoeopathic Remedies
for
Women's Ailments

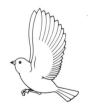

Health Science Press
The C. W. Daniel Company Ltd
1 Church Path, Saffron Walden, Essex, England

Other books by Phyllis Speight
Arnica the Wonder Herb
Before Calling the Doctor
Comparison of the Chronic Miasms
Homoeopathy – A Practical Guide to Natural Medicine
Overcoming Rheumatism and Arthritis
Pertinent Questions and Answers about Homoeopathy
A Study Course in Homoeopathy
Homoeopathic Remedies for Children
Homoeopathy for Emergencies

Reprinted 1988

ISBN 0 85032 200 6

Set in 10pt Photina, 2pt leaded and printed in
Great Britain by White Crescent Press Ltd,
Luton, Bedfordshire

CONTENTS

PREFACE

Many women have come to see me suffering from troublesome periods, feeling unwell during the menopause or a difficult pregnancy and I have always been surprised at their attitudes because most of them convey the idea that every woman suffers at these particular times.

'It's my age, of course', this has been said to me literally dozens of times and I have felt, sometimes, that some women would be disappointed if they didn't have anything to complain about during the menopause.

Puberty, when the monthly periods commence, childbirth and the menopause are all natural functions and women who are happy and healthy have little or no trouble.

But we are living in an age of sophistication when equality of the sexes encourages many more women to work. Life seems to have speeded up, there is never enough time; tensions and strains become part of the general life-style and often the inevitable tranquillizers and sleeping pills follow. Meals have to be prepared quickly, hence the demand for convenience foods, packaged and tinned, containing additives, colouring, preservatives and all kinds of things which are harmful.

This book is written with the idea of not only helping but re-educating; it is never too late to learn, and we can all change our ways if we really wish to do so.

I sincerely hope that very many women of all ages will benefit from this book by becoming more happy and more healthy people.

Phyllis Speight
Devon, 1985

INTRODUCTION

Homoeopathy is a complete system of medicine which has been in use since the early 1800s.

It is based on the Law of Similars which means that a remedy which will produce symptoms when taken by healthy people will cure similar symptoms in sick people – *Similia Similibus Curantur*, let like be cured by like.

In order to find out what symptoms remedies will cure, each one has been 'proved' on healthy men and women. In other words they took a remedy, under the supervision of a doctor, and after a while symptoms were produced. These were carefully noted and collated and form the materia medica from which we work today.

We treat patients by matching their symptoms to those produced by the remedy.

For instance *Pulsatilla* produced symptoms that are always changing, pains move from joint to joint, periods change in appearance and the disposition changes from laughter to tears. Heat cannot be tolerated and there is a craving for fresh air. Fats and fatty foods are not tolerated. This, of course, is very brief, but a patient suffering from changeable periods with other matching symptoms, will be cured by *Pulsatilla*.

The following pages should be studied carefully in order that the most similar remedy to the patients' symptoms may be found.

With patience and care many troubles can be dealt with successfully, but in a book of this size the number of remedies has to be limited. If, therefore, there is little or no improvement within a reasonable time, then the skills of an experienced homoeopath should be sought, because, sometimes, what appears to be something quite simple could prove to be rather more serious than originally suspected.

NOTES ON THE 38 REMEDIES

In each of the 38 remedies I have commenced by giving the characteristic symptoms. These are the most important because they are the core and 'individualize' each remedy.

The characteristic symptoms are followed by: Anxiety and fear; Breasts; Constipation; Cystitis; Depression; Diarrhoea; Haemorrhoids; Headache; Leucorrhoea; Menopause; Menses; Metrorrhagia; Miscarriage; Pregnancy; Pre-menstrual tension; Sexual intercourse; Sleeplessness; Sterility; Subinvolution; Uterus; Vagina; Varicose ulcer; Varicose veins, Vulva.

A word or two about some of these symptoms. Most are quite straightforward but under Breasts I have included any trouble that may occur during menses and, of course, during pregnancy; mastitis comes under this heading.

Constipation is very common and when chronic there is always toxic absorption. More serious troubles can develop and it is wise to eliminate the condition rather than take laxatives every night. They will never cure constipation and in the end the bowel becomes lazy. The chapter on diet should be of help.

I have included diarrhoea mainly because if it develops during pregnancy it could lead to an abortion if not cleared up quickly.

Metrorrhagia is bleeding from the uterus at times other than at the monthly periods and should be cleared up as soon as possible.

It should be emphasized that all irregular uterine bleeding before, during or after the menopause must always be fully investigated, and not just attributed to the menopause.

Subinvolution is failure of the lately pregnant uterus to return to its normal size within the usual time of 6 weeks.

You will notice that all the headings are not included under every remedy, this is because those omitted were not brought out in the provings.

Also, I have listed only the symptoms which will help in

diseases of women, many more under each remedy are omitted.

And finally, there are many more remedies which have cured the diseases mentioned but in a book of this size the number had to be limited and I have tried to choose those most constantly called for.

HOW TO CHOOSE THE CORRECT REMEDY

The 38 remedies should be studied very carefully and I would suggest that the characteristic symptoms are memorized because this would make the task of finding the correct remedy much easier.

The first step is to write down all the symptoms. The important things to know are how the person feels; the location of the pain; what the pain is like, eg sore, stabbing, throbbing, burning, etc; what makes it better or worse, and the cause, if known.

It is always much more difficult to treat oneself, we cannot see ourselves objectively enough, but if there is no alternative then the questions must be answered truthfully and with care.

When all the answers are written down, then the most similar remedy must be chosen.

To make this a little easier I have included a repertory. This gives all the remedies from the 38 that have 'Anxiety and fear'; all that have symptoms under 'Breast' and so on.

Then follows a repertory of the mental characteristic symptoms and then the physical characteristic symptoms – these are in alphabetical order so that any characteristic symptom may be found quickly.

Modalities follow giving all the situations that make the patient feel worse, and better.

And then there is a General repertory which lists the symptoms and remedies under each section, e.g. symptoms of diarrhoea from all remedies which include diarrhoea.

All these lists are for reference and can be very helpful.

If you have three or more characteristic symptoms that are marked in the sick person then there is no doubt that you will find other matching symptoms and the remedy may be given with confidence because, as I have said before, the characteristic symptoms are the most important.

REMEDIES AND THEIR ABBREVIATIONS

Aconite	Acon.
Alumina	Alum.
Apis Mellifica	Apis.
Arnica Montana	Arn.
Arsenicum Album	Ars.
Belladonna	Bell.
Borax	Bor.
Bryonia	Bry.
Calcarea Carbonica	Calc.
Caulophyllum	Caul.
Causticum	Caust.
Chamomilla	Cham.
China (Cinchona)	China.
Cimicifuga	Cim.
Cocculus	Cocc.
Conium	Con.
Gelsemium	Gels.
Graphites	Graph.
Ipecacuanha	Ip.
Kali Carbonica	Kali C.
Kreosote	Kreos.
Lachesis	Lach.
Lilium Tigrinum	Lil T.
Lycopodium	Lyc.
Mercurius Solubilis	Merc.
Natrum Muriaticum	Nat M.
Nitric Acid	Nit Ac.
Nux Moschata	Nux M.
Nux Vomica	Nux V.
Phosphorus	Phos.
Platinum	Plat.
Podophyllum	Pod.

REMEDIES AND THEIR ABBREVIATIONS

Pulsatilla	Puls.
Sabina	Sab.
Secale Cornutum	Sec.
Sepia	Sep.
Silica	Sil.
Sulphur	Sul.

HOMOEOPATHIC REMEDIES

Homoeopathic remedies are prepared in a special way by Homoeopathic Chemists and should always be purchased from a reliable firm.

They are sensitive and should be kept in a drawer or cupboard away from sunlight and strong smelling perfumes or soaps etc, and they should not be taken directly after cleaning the teeth with a flavoured toothpaste.

Pills or tablets should be handled as little as possible – usually they can be shaken into the cap of the bottle or box and popped into the mouth.

One pill or tablet is sufficient for one dose. Put one or the other under the tongue where it will dissolve – do NOT wash it down with water.

In acute troubles remedies may be given frequently in the 6th or 12th potencies – half-hourly if necessary but usually one or two hourly is adequate – this depends entirely how severe the condition is. The golden rule is that as improvement develops the time between doses must be widened and the medicine stopped as soon as the patient is much better – remedies continue to work in the system for some time after the last dose has been taken.

If similar symptoms return then the remedy may be repeated but if new symptoms appear then a different remedy must be found to match them.

If after a day the patient is not improving another must be found to match the symptoms more accurately. Do NOT change the remedy too quickly. This emphasizes the importance of finding the correct remedy.

If there is no sign of improvement or the condition gets worse then a doctor must be consulted at once.

ACONITE

Characteristics:

Fear, anxiety, physical and mental restlessness.
Fright – Aconite has a calming effect.
The sudden beginning of an acute illness with fever, anxiety, restlessness and fear.
Fearful of the future, of death, there are so many fears.
Can vomit with fear.
There is much tension.
Complaints caused by exposure to dry cold winds and weather.
Worse: Warm room; around midnight; cold dry winds.
Better: Open air.

Anxiety and Fear: Fear will often cause inflammation of uterus or ovaries in excitable women.
It will also cause or threaten miscarriage. Aconite given early will check this.
Fear of dying in confinement.
Fearful after labour.
Palpitation with great anxiety.
Extreme fearfulness.

Headaches: Can be extremely violent.
Tearing, burning in brain with fear, fever and anguish.
Fullness and heaviness in forehead.
Throbbing in left side of forehead.

Leucorrhoea: Copious, tenacious, yellowish.

Menopause: With flushes of heat.

Menses (Periods): Generally too late, diminished, but too protracted.
Suppressed by fright.

Miscarriage: Threatened from fright.
With fever, restlessness, thirst, dry skin, anxiety and fear.

Ovaries: Congested and painful.

Pre-Menstrual Tension: Nervous, restless.

Pregnancy: During – restless, fearful, fears death.
Labour pains sharp, violent, rapid.
Parts dry, tender. Contractions insufficient.
After pains too painful, last too long.

Sleeplessness: Restless, excited, tossing about, fearful.
Especially useful after chill, shock, fright – Aconite will give peace and sleep.

Uterus: Prolapse, sudden with inflammation.

Vagina: Dry, hot, sensitive.
Inflammation.

ALUMINA

Characteristics:

Hasty, hurried, time passes too slowly.
Variable mood, better as day advances.
Dryness of mucous membranes. Sluggish functions.
Abnormal cravings for chalk, charcoal, coffee grounds, indigestible things.
Worse: Morning; warm room.
Better: Open air and damp weather.

Constipation: Inactivity of rectum. Must strain even for soft stools.
Rectum seems paralysed; no strength to push contents out.
Stools hard, knotty like sheep's dung with cutting at anus; or soft like clay.

Diarrhoea: With urging in rectum when urinating.
Clots of blood pass from anus.

Haemorrhoids: Itching and burning; worse evening.
Better after a night's rest.

Leucorrhoea: Acrid, profuse, ropy with burning.
Worse daytime.
Relieved by washing in cold water.

Menses (Periods): Too early, scanty, pale, followed by great exhaustion.
Often preceded by headache.

Pre-Menstrual Tension: Weakness.

Vagina: Clear discharge with burning and itching. Painful throbbing on left side.

Vulva: Sore and often itching.

APIS MELLIFICA

Characteristics:

> Jealous and suspicious.
> Whining; tearfulness.
> Awkward, often drops things.
> Constricted sensations.
> Oedema.
> Pains stinging and burning.
> Alternately dry and hot or perspiring.
> Thirstlessness; sweats without thirst.
> Cannot stand heat; warm room, hot bath.
> Better: Cold room, cold air, cold applications.

Constipation: Bowels seem to be paralysed. No stool for days, even a week. Feels as if something would break on straining.

Cystitis: Agony in voiding urine. Frequent, painful, scanty, bloody urination. Only a few drops after straining. Urine almost suppressed.
Pain in region of bladder.
Retention when nursing infants.

Depression: With constant weeping without cause.
Premonition of death.
Mental and all symptoms worse in warm room.

Diarrhoea: Watery, yellow with griping. Watery and foul smelling.
Greenish yellow with mucus. Slimy mucus and blood.
Frequent bloody, painless diarrhoea.
Worse morning. Extreme weakness.

Haemorrhoids: With stinging pain, especially after confinement.

Headaches: Pain in occiput, occasionally sharp.
Pains like bee-stings followed by burning.

Menses (Periods): Excessive flow with heaviness in abdomen.
Faintness, uneasiness, restlessness.
Painful periods with scanty discharge of slimy blood.
Periods absent.

Miscarriage: During early months, around second month.
Tendency to.

Ovaries: Congestion, feeling of weight and heaviness.
Enlarged.
Inflammation.
Pains; burning, especially after intercourse.
Lancinating and stinging.

Uterus: Inflammation.

ARNICA MONTANA

Characteristics:

> In serious illness says there is nothing the matter with her.
> After traumatic injuries.
> Sore, lame bruised feeling.
> Worse: Cold, damp.

Anxiety and Fear: Anxious about herself; no doctor can help.
Attacks of anxiety.
Apprehension about the future.
Fear of being approached.
Fearful dreams.
Restless because everything she lies on is too hard.

Breasts: Mastitis from injury.
Nipples sore.

Cystitis: After mechanical injuries.
Constant urging whilst urine passes in drops.
Frequent attempts to urinate, has to wait a long time for it to pass.
Urine can be thick with pus.

Headaches: Burning in head whilst rest of body is cool.
Aching pains over eyes to temples.
Shooting in head from coughing, sneezing.
Cutting pain in head then coldness.
Effects of injuries to head; concussion.

Miscarriage: From injuries.

Pregnancy: The great remedy after delivery, for relief and comfort and to avoid sepsis.
Bruised parts after labour.
Violent after-pains.

Sleeplessness: Too tired to sleep.
Bed feels too hard; part laid on too sore – must move for relief.
Sleeplessness after exertion and physical strain.

Varicose Ulcers: During pregnancy.

Varicose Veins: During pregnancy.

ARSENICUM ALBUM

Characteristics:

Great anguish and restlessness.
Fear, fright and worry.
Prostration yet marked restlessness from anxiety making patient change places constantly.
Great exhaustion after slightest exertion.
Fastidious, hates disorder.
Burning pains better by heat but patient always wants the head kept cool.
Burning discharges.
Great thirst for small quantities at frequent intervals.
Worse: Cold air; wet weather; cold drinks; cold applications; night, after midnight, 1 am to 3 am.
Better: Warmth (except head). Loves and craves heat.

Anxiety and Fear: Intense anxiety in pregnancy with fear; of being alone; of death; that something terrible is going to happen. This anxiety brings restlessness yet she cannot rest anywhere. Excessive anxiety.
Anxiety and restlessness indescribable.

Breasts: Nipples burning; cracked.

Constipation: With pain in bowels.

Depression: Weary of life, dread of death when alone or on going to bed.
Despair of recovery.
Melancholy.

Diarrhoea: Painless, offensive, watery stools.
Diarrhoea and constipation often alternate.

Haemorrhoids: Stitching pain while walking and sitting but not at stool.
Burning pains in anus better heat.
Haemorrhoids protrude like coals of fire.

Headaches: Periodic every few days.
Wants head cool while rest of body well wrapped up. Head better bathed with cold water.
Congestive, throbs and burns.
Headaches with nausea and vomiting.
Very bad sick headaches with thirst, little and often.
Very bad occipital headaches – begin after midnight; from excitement; feels dazed.
Any neuralgic headache needing this remedy wants the head kept warm.

Leucorrhoea: Yellow, acrid, excoriating; profuse; thick and corroding.

Menses (Periods): Too early, too profuse.
Excessive flow exhausting.
Painful.
Scanty, pale periods.
Thin, whitish, offensive discharge instead of period.

Ovaries: Pain, burning; drawing worse motion.
Stitching, right ovary.

Pregnancy: Involuntary urination.
Persistent vomiting in spite of sips of water – state of dehydration with great weakness but also anxious and restless.

Sleeplessness: With restlessness, moaning, tossing, uneasiness after midnight.
Attacks of anxiety drive her out of bed.
From muscular exertion.

Varicose Ulcer: On legs, deep, painful, burning, could become gangrenous.

Varicose Veins: During pregnancy.

Uterus: Polypus.

BELLADONNA

Characteristics:

This remedy stands for HEAT, REDNESS, THROBBING and BURNING.

Attacks are violent and onset sudden.

Many acute local inflammations; fevers with hot, burning, dry skin, so hot that heat can be felt by the hand before it touches the skin.

Very red, flushed face; dilated pupils of the eyes.

Sudden rise in temperature.

Restless sleep from excited mental states which can go on to delirium.

There is often an acuteness of all senses.

Can get very angry.

Anxiety and Fear: Fears imaginary things, wants to escape; run away.

Starts in fright when approached.

Great anxiety, must go away.

Breasts: Swelling; sore.

Lactation, too copious milk flow.

Inflammation of breasts; they are red, hot, swollen and very tender.

Breasts dry, stony-hard, very tender.

Mastitis.

Cystitis: Great irritation of bladder; constant urging to urinate.

Dribbling urine, burns intensely.

Bladder sensitive to jar and pressure.

Urine bloody or little clots.

Urine can be very acid. Sometimes fiery red.

Headaches: Violent; congestion, red, hot face, throbbing, cutting, shooting and stabbing pain.
Every step jars.
Bursting pain, worse stooping.
Worse noise, jar, motion, light, lying down, better pressure.
Violent headache, better drawing head back.
Headache with dizziness, worse stooping.
Headache from washing head.
Headaches come suddenly, last an indefinite time, and then depart suddenly.

Menopause: With flushes of heat.

Menses (Periods): Bright red, sometimes mingled with clots.
Dark, with sudden clots.
Copious; too frequent, too early, too soon.
Offensive; painful; suppressed.
Congestion of uterus during periods.

Miscarriage:

Metrorrhagia (Bleeding from Uterus): When physically active.
Coagulated, with clots.
Profuse; sudden.

Ovaries: Enlarged; inflammation.
Pain in right ovary worse motion.

Sleeplessness: Cannot sleep in spite of feeling sleepy.
Restless with frightful dreams.
Uneasy sleep before midnight.

Subinvolution: If other symptoms agree this remedy will help.

Uterus: Displacement of.
Inflammation.
Pain: Bearing down pains in uterus region as if everything would come out; worse morning.
Pains constrictive, drawing and griping.
Pains during menses, paroxysmal, worse motion.
Labour pains false.
Pain pinching while walking. Pressing.
Sore and tenderness, worse motion.
Sensitive to jarring.
Pain stitching.
Polypus.

BORAX

Characteristics:

Dread of downward motion in nearly all complaints, which brings anxiety.
Very nervous and frightened.
Sensitive to sudden noise.
Worse: Warm weather.
Better: Cold weather.

Anxiety and Fear: A great dread of downward motion; afraid of going downstairs; cannot swing or use a rocking chair.
Child screams on waking and grasps sides of cradle or pram.
Easily startled.
Sensitive, nervous, fidgety.

Leucorrhoea: Like the white of an egg: excoriating, burning.
Acrid discharge midway between periods.

Menopause: With flushes of heat.

Menses (Periods): Too early, too profuse, with colic, griping and nausea.
Feels worse after periods.

Sterility: If other symptoms agree this remedy will help.

Vagina: General soreness and itching.
Hot, smarting pains in urinary orifice.

Vulva: Pruritis, itching.

BRYONIA

Characteristics:

Complaints develop slowly.
Great irritability. Don't cross a Bryonia patient, it makes him worse.
Excessive thirst for copious draughts at long intervals.
Stitching and tearing pains which are worse for any movement and better for rest.
Dryness of mucous membranes from lips to rectum.
Faintness when head is raised (sitting up in bed).
The Bryonia patient is worse from the slightest movement; and is worse from warmth.
Better: Pressure, lying on painful side; cold things.
(In a damp climate Bryonia is required very frequently.)

Anxiety and Fear: About the future! Great sense of insecurity. Worried about her business.

Breasts: Swollen, sore, painful with periods.
Mastitis.

Constipation: Chronic with severe headache.
No desire; urging with several attempts before results.
Stools hard, dark, dry, seem too large after straining.
After stool, long continued burning in rectum.

Diarrhoea: Preceded by cutting pains in abdomen.
Bilious, acrid stools with soreness of anus.
Stools like dirty water with whitish granulated sediments of undigestible food.
Urging followed by copious, pasty evacuations.
Diarrhoea with relief of all symptoms except confusion of head.

Headaches: Worse from any motion, needs to be perfectly still and not disturbed mentally or emotionally.
Bursting, splitting or crushing headache.
Nausea or faintness on rising or sitting up.
Grasps head when about to cough.

Menses (Periods): Too early, too profuse; suppressed with frequent bleeding of nose.
Brown, offensive.

Ovaries: Sore or stitching pains worse motion; walking.

Pre-Menstrual Tension: Stomach disturbance, headache.

Sleeplessness: Very restless, waking sometimes every half hour.
Mind active.
Sleeplessness before midnight.
Delusion that she is away and wants to go home.

Uterus: Sore pains, worse walking and motion.

CALCAREA CARBONICA

Characteristics:

Fat, flabby, fair, faint.
A jaded state, mental or physical due to overwork.
Apprehensive and fearful.
Hand is soft, cool and boneless; gives you the shivers to shake hands with Calcarea.
Everything smells sour, stool, sweat, urine, and taste is sour.
Profuse cold, sour sweat, especially on head.
Sweats even in cold room.
Enlargement of glands.
Slow in movement.
Craves eggs and indigestible things like chalk, earth, raw potatoes.
Feels better when constipated.
Feet feel as if wearing cold, damp stockings.
Great sensitivity to cold, and cold, damp weather; dreads open air; at the same time cannot bear the sun.
Breathless; walking slowly up a slight hill can bring on sweating and breathlessness.
Worse: On waking; morning; after midnight; bathing; working in water; full moon; new moon; mental and physical exertion; stooping; pressure of clothes; open air; cold air; cold wet weather; letting limbs hang down.
Better: After breakfast; drawing up limbs; loosening garments; in the dark; lying on back; from rubbing; dry, warm weather.

Anxiety and Fear: Calcarea has every kind of fear.
Thinks about imaginery things that might happen to her.
Great anxiety with palpitation.
Mind is uneasy; wondering what will happen to her; expecting bad news; dreading the future.
Easily frightened – has so many fears.

Breasts: Soreness.

Lactation, profuse secretion of watery milk which the child refuses.

Excessive lactation with fever, sweat and debility.

Breasts distended, milk scanty.

Cold, feels cold air.

Milk disagrees.

Milk has a disagreeable, nauseating taste, child will not nurse and cries.

Hot swelling of breasts.

Constipation: Stubborn; stool chalky white.

Patient usually feels better when constipated.

Hard, difficult, clay-coloured stools.

Undigested stool often with slime, smelling like bad eggs.

Diarrhoea: Frequent, first hard then pasty, then liquid, thin, offensive; yellowish, grey or clay-like. Whitish, watery; worse afternoon or evening. Sour smelling.

Haemorrhoids: Protruding, painful when walking, better sitting.

Painful, bleeding.

Intense aching and shooting in rectum hours after stool.

Headaches: Icy coldness in and on top of head.

Pressive pain and heaviness in forehead.

Tearing headache above eyes.

Head feels numb as if wearing a cap.

Leucorrhoea: Burning, gushing, copious before, after and between menses, milky, thick.

Itching with burning.

Menopause: With flooding, bleeding between period time and flushes of heat which travel upwards.

Menses (Periods): Clotted, copious after excitement or exertion.

Frequent, protracted; worse mental excitement.

Metrorrhagia (Bleeding from Uterus): Between periods, at menopause; after exertion; profuse.

Miscarriage: Tendency to.

Pre-Menstrual Tension: Depression, giddy feeling.

Sexual Desire: Increased.

Sleeplessness: Many thoughts crowd into mind, or thoughts go round and round.
Cold feet at night in bed.
Head sweats in sleep.

Subinvolution: If other symptoms agree this remedy will help.

Uterus: Pain before and during periods.
Labour pains false.
Fibroids.
Displacement.
Polypus.

Vagina: Itching.
Polypus.

Varicose Ulcer: Deep.

Varicose Veins: Inflamed.

Vulva: Violent itching and soreness, inflammation and swelling.

CAULOPHYLLUM

Characteristics:

> A woman's remedy.
> Want of tonicity of uterus.

Leucorrhoea: Profuse; mucus.

Menses (Periods): Too soon, profuse; painful colic.

Miscarriage: Habitual from uterus debility.

Pre-Menstrual Tension: Hysteria.

Subinvolution: If other symptoms agree this remedy will help.

Uterus: Cramping pains before menses.
Labour pains false.
Labour pains short, irregular, spasmodic.
Contractions spasmodic.
Sensation of congestion.
After-pains spasmodic.
Retroverted.

Vagina: Irritable, spasmodic, intense pains.
Ulceration.

CAUSTICUM

Characteristics:

Intensely sympathetic.
Depression, apprehension, timidity, irritability.
Aches and pains with soreness, rawness and burning.
Paralysis of single parts, e.g. face, throat, vocal chords, limbs, from exposure to cold, dry winds.
Skin dirty white, sallow.
Worse: Dry, cold winds in fine, clear weather. Cold air.
Better: Damp, wet weather; warmth.

Breasts: Nipples cracked, sore, surrounded with herpes.

Constipation: Often ineffectual efforts to stool with anxiety, pain and red face.
Inaction of rectum; gets full of hard faeces which pass unnoticed.
Little balls are passed unnoticed.
Stool tough and slimy like grease.
Stools passed better when standing.

Cystitis: Frequent urging through the 24 hours.
Ineffectual attempts to urinate; pain in bladder after a few drops.
Has to wait a long time then very little is passed and there is urging once more without pain.
Pain retention from cold.
Itching of urethral office.

Haemorrhoids: Impede stool; swollen, itching, stitching, moist; stinging, burning, painful when touched, when walking or when thinking of them.

Leucorrhoea: Profuse, flows like period and has same odour.
Only at Night.

Menopause: With flushes of heat, followed by chilliness.

Menses (Periods): Too early, too profuse and after ceasing a little is passed from time to time for days.
Sometimes large clots.
Bad odour.
Excites itching in vulva.
Stop at night.

Pregnancy: Depression.
After labour when it has been long and slow.
Overstretched bladder.

Pre-Menstrual Tension: With depression.

Sexual Desire: Diminished.
Aversion to.
Enjoyment absent.

Uterus: Labour pains spasmodic.
Inertia during labour.

Vagina: Itching.

Varicose Veins: Painful.

CHAMOMILLA

Characteristics:

Frantic, irritability – cannot bear it – whatever it may be!
Impatient, over-sensitive.
Whining restlessness; impatient, snappish.
Is bad tempered when she cannot get what she wants.
Inability to control temper.
Worse: Heat.
Better: Warm, wet weather.

Breasts: Sore.
Mastitis.
Nipples cracked, sore, inflamed, tender to touch.
Can hardly bear the pain of nursing.

Cystitis: Sticking pain in neck of bladder when not urinating.
Ineffectual urging with anguish.
Burning pain when urinating.
Urine hot, scanty, turbid, blood-red.

Diarrhoea: Watery, frequent, preceded by cutting, constricting tummy-ache.
Mucus with colic and vomiting.
Burning in anus, painful, thin, green stools with faeces and mucus.
Green watery stools corroding, with colic; thirst, bitter taste and bitter eructations.

Leucorrhoea: Yellow, acrid and excoriating.

Menses (Periods): Frequent, dark, clotted, membranous and painful.

Metrorrhagia (Bleeding from Uterus): Bleeding from uterus after anger.
Coagulated.

Pre-Menstrual Tension: Nervous, restless, irritability.

Sleeplessness: Sleepy but cannot get to sleep.
Restless, especially early at night.
As soon as bedtime comes is wide awake.
Violent pains come on in night preventing sleep.

Uterine Haemorrhages: Profuse discharge of dark blood with labour pains.
After pains.

Uterus: Bearing down pains.
Pains cramping, after anger. Paroxysmal.
Pains cramping before and during periods.
Pains griping, labour-like during periods.
Labour pains distressing, excessive, spasmodic.

CHINA (CINCHONA)

Characteristics:

Debility and complaints after excessive loss of fluids: bleeding; periods; diarrhoea.
Haemorrhage can be profuse with fainting.
Periodical affections, especially every other day.
Worse: Slight touch; least draught of air.
Better: Hard pressure on painful part; open air; warmth.

Depression: Apathetic, indifferent, taciturn.
Worn down by exhausting discharges.
No desire to live.
Extreme sensitiveness; cannot bear noise or excitement.
Extreme nervous irritability.

Diarrhoea: Loose, brownish, painless, with feeling of debility.
Frothy, painless stools with fermentation in bowels.
Offensive undigested or white papescent stools at night; yellow, watery, involuntary.
Diarrhoea comes on gradually, getting more and more watery, pale, pinkish, with rapid emaciation.

Headaches: Congestive, extremities covered in cold sweat.
Stitching pain from temple to temple.
Pains from occiput over whole head.
Intense throbbing.
Feels as if head would burst.
Worse: Draught.
Better: From hard pressure.

Leucorrhoea: Bloody. Seems to take the place of the usual menstrual discharge.

Menses (Periods): Copious. Dark clots and abdominal distention.

Metrorrhagia (Bleeding from Uterus): Dark blood.

Ovaries: Feel heavy.

CIMICIFUGA

Characteristics:

> Agitation and pain indicate this remedy.
> The greater the flow, the greater the pain.
> Great depression with dream of impending evil.
> Worse: Cold.
> Better: Warmth.

Anxiety and Fear: Fearful in pregnancy.

Depression: Sensation of heavy cloud settling on her.
Feels confused with weight on head.
Grieved, troubled, sighing.
Mind disturbed by disappointed love or business failure.

Menopause: With flooding, flushing, headaches and mental depression.

Menses (Periods): Feels worse during periods.
Pain immediately before period.
Profuse, dark, coagulated, offensive, with backache. Always irregular.
Sharp pains across abdomen, has to double up; labour like pains.
Debility between periods.

Miscarriage: Tendency to.

Pregnancy: Labour pains weak, ceasing; severe, tedious, weak or spasmodic with faintness or cramps.
Nausea; false, labour-like pains.
Sharp pains across abdomen.
Sleeplessness.
After pains with great sensitiveness and intolerance of pain: nausea and vomiting.

43

Pre-Menstrual Tension: Nervous, restless, headache, depression.

Subinvolution: If other symptoms agree this remedy will help.

Uterus: Stitching pains from side to side.
Bearing down pains.
Great tenderness in this region.

COCCULUS

Characteristics:

Extreme irritability of nervous system.
Cannot bear contradiction.
Profound sadness.
Effects of night-watching.
Sensation of hollowness – emptiness.
Time passes too quickly. Slowness in thinking, worse after an emotional disturbance.
Sensitive to hot or cold air.

Constipation: Rectum paralysed; inability to press at stool or to evacuate.
Inability to use muscles of evacuation.
Feels awful after stool and sometimes faints.

Headaches: As if skull would burst.
Sick headaches with giddy feeling.
Thought or smell of food nauseates.
Travel sickness with headache and nausea.
On motion eyes feel as if being torn from sockets.
Pulsating pains on top of head and in temples.
Headache at nape of neck and back of head as if opening and shutting.
Worse: Eating, drinking, sleeping.
Better: Rest, indoors.

Leucorrhoea: Gushing, purulent, between periods.
Very weakening.

Menses (Periods): Too frequent, too early, too soon.
Copious, worse standing, and walking.
Pain cramping, cutting; colic.
Very weak during periods.

Pre-Menstrual Tension: Weakness, headaches, irritability, depression.

Sleeplessness: From vexation, grief, anxiety and prolonged loss of sleep.
Exhausted but cannot sleep.
Ill effects from long nursing.

Uterus: Pains cutting, worse motion.

CONIUM

Characteristics:

Dizziness, numbness, paralytic weakness, mental and physical.
Weakness of body and mind, trembling.
Sweats copiously during sleep or merely closing the eyes.

Breasts: Enlarge and become painful before and during periods.
Lax and shrunken, painful to touch.
Mastitis.
Nipples burning; sore; stitching pain.

Constipation: Ineffectual urging, hard stool, small quantities passed each time.
Inability to strain at stool.
Burning in rectum during stool.
After stool trembling and weakness.

Menses (Periods): Late, scanty, suppressed, absent.

Ovaries: Enlarged; inflammation.

Pre-Menstrual Tension: Depression.

Sexual Desire: Increased.

Uterus: Enlarged.
Polypus.

Vagina: Itching.

GELSEMIUM

Characteristics:

Affects more the nerves of motion, causing muscular prostration and varying degrees of motor paralysis.
Dizziness, drowsiness, dullness, trembling.
Tiredness, limbs feel tired; eyelids feel heavy.
Fearful; terrors of anticipation.
Apathy regarding illness.
Worse: Damp weather; emotion; excitement; bad news; 10 am.
Better: Bending forward; open air; continued motion. Headache is relieved by profuse urination.

Anxiety and Fear: Bad effects of great fright or fear.
Anticipation brings on diarrhoea.
Tremor; wants to be held – lacks courage; wants to be alone.

Headaches: Congestive; most violent at back of head.
Hammering at base of brain.
Lies high and exhausted with pain.
Later whole head congested; really dreadful pain, eyes glassy, pupils dilated. Extremities cold.
Or neuralgic headache in temples and over eyes, with nausea and vomiting.
Headaches relieved by copious urination.

Menses (Periods): Painful with scanty flow.

Miscarriage: From fright.

Pregnancy: Griping, labour-like.
Distressing, spasmodic labour pains.
False labour pains.
Labour pains weak.
Rigidity of Os.

Pre-Menstrual Tension: Headache.

GRAPHITES

Characteristics:

Has an affinity with women who are overweight, chilly and constipated.
Obesity.
Music causes patient to cry.
Intolerance of light, especially sunlight.
Very rough skin with cracks.
Eruptions oozing sticky, honey-like substance.
Always cold but craves fresh air, must be well wrapped up.
On the other hand she suffers when the weather is very hot.
Worse: Warmth; at night.
Better: In the dark; wrapping up.

Anxiety and Fear: Timid, unable to make decisions.
Apprehensive, indecisive.
Great tendency to stare.
Fidgets while sitting.

Breasts: Swelling; hardness.
Nipples cracked, sore and blistered.

Constipation: Stool large, hard, knotty, in masses with tough, slimy mucus.
There can be much mucus with hard stool.

Haemorrhoids: Large, with pain on sitting, or on taking a wide step as if split with a knife; also violent itching and very sore to touch.

Leucorrhoea: Acrid, excoriating, copious; thin, watery, white.
Gushing before menses.
Great weakness.

Menopause: Rush of blood to head, and heat of face.
Nose bleed.

Menses (Periods): Late, pale, scanty.
Suppressed.
Absent.
First period delayed in girls.
Cramping pains during period.
Feels worse during period.
Itching before menses.

Ovaries: Stitching pain.

Pre-Menstrual Tension: Headache.
Weakness.

Sexual Intercourse: Aversion to.

Uterus: Cramping pain.

Vagina: Itching.

Varicose Veins: During pregnancy.

Varicose Ulcers: In foot.
In legs.
In toes, originating in blisters.

IPECACUANHA

Characteristics:

Persistent nausea. Nausea unrelieved by vomiting.
Nausea and vomiting with clean tongue.
Haemorrhage bright red and profuse.
Peevish, irritable, impatient, scornful.
Ailments from vexation.

Diarrhoea: With much pain.
Stools yellow, painless, fermented; green as grass with nausea and colic; green mucus; covered with red, bloody mucus.
Autumnal diarrhoea with griping.

Menses (Periods): Bright red, clotted, copious with faintness; too early, too frequent.

Metrorrhagia (Bleeding from Uterus): Bleeding between periods when active; bright red, gushing worse motion.
During and after labour, profuse.

Pregnancy: Morning sickness with much nausea.

Uterus: Haemorrhage profuse, bright, gushing with nausea.
Pain from navel to uterus.

KALI CARBONICUM

Characteristics:

Very irritable.
Anxiety felt in the stomach.
Hypersensitive to pain, noise and touch.
All pains are sharp cutting.
Stitches may be felt in any part of the body.
Intolerance of cold weather.
Worse: From soup and coffee; at 3 am; lying on left and painful side.
Better: Warm, moist weather; moving about.

Anxiety and Fear: About her disease; that she cannot recover.
Frightened if anything touches the body lightly, hates to be touched.
Shocks are felt in the stomach.
Great aversion to being alone.

Leucorrhoea: Yellow with backache; labour-like pains.
Itching and burning in vulva from discharges.

Menopause: With flushing; loss of appetite, biliousness, taste of bile in mouth on waking.

Menses (Periods): Too frequent, too early, pale, scanty, acrid; flow may be early, more profuse and longer lasting than usual.
Painful.
Absent.
Delayed in girls (first period); difficult first period.

Miscarriage: Tendency to, especially around second month.

Pre-Menstrual Tension: Feels worse before and during periods but better afterwards.
Stomach disturbance.

Sleeplessness: Drowsy after eating.
Wakes up about 2 am and cannot sleep afterwards.

Uterus: Pain before period.
Pain griping, labour like.
Labour pains distressing, weak.
Labour pains ceasing.
After pains.

Varicose Ulcers: In legs.

Vagina: Itching.

KREOSOTE

Characteristics:

Stupid; forgetful, peevish, irritable.
Excoriating and offensive discharges.
Worse: Open air; cold; rest; when lying; after menstruation.
Better: Warmth; motion; warm food.

Leucorrhoea: Acrid, excoriating; burning (before periods); yellow; putrid in pregnancy.
Itching.

Menses (Periods): Intermits, flow ceases on sitting or walking, reappears on lying down.
Offensive; too early; prolonged.
Difficult hearing during periods.
Pains worse after periods.

Metrorrhagia (Bleeding from Uterus): After sexual intercourse.

Pregnancy: Vomiting.

Pre-Menstrual Tension: Feels worse before and during periods.
Irritable, nervous, restless headaches.

Uterus: Bearing down pain as if everything would come down.
Biting, burning pain worse while and after urinating.
Sore, tender.

Vagina: Itching, voluptuous; sore, tender.
Violent itching, worse urinating.

Varicose Veins: Lower limbs.

Vulva: Corrosive itching; burning and soreness.

LACHESIS

Characteristics:

Insanely jealous and suspicious.
Loquacity.
Worse from sleep. Sleeps into an aggravation (no matter what the symptoms).
Worse left side. Sometimes moving to the right.
Intolerance of anything tight, especially round neck or waist.
Worse: After sleep; left side; in the spring; pressure or constriction; hot drinks.
Better: Warm applications; the appearance of any discharge.

Anxiety and Fear: Fear of death, of being poisoned.
Full of anxiety, worse waking.

Breasts: Sore.
Mastitis.

Constipation: Costive; ineffectual urging; anus feels closed.
Thin offensive stools.
Beating in anus as if from hammers.

Cystitis: With offensive mucus, 'the more offensiveness the more it is Lachesis'.
Can hardly bear to let clothes touch abdomen.
Urine blackish or dark brown; foamy.
Ineffectual urging; violent burning when it does pass.
No urine, no stool.
Always has to urinate after lying down and especially after sleep.

Diarrhoea: Diarrhoea and constipation in alternation.
Stools watery, light yellow or dark chocolate coloured, foul smelling.
Worse at night, after acids, during warm weather.

Haemorrhoids: Protruding or strangulated or with stitches upward at each cough or sneeze.
Itching at anus.

Headaches: Violent congestion with vomiting.
Throbbing, bursting pain as if all the blood of body had gone to head.
Chronic headaches whenever exposed to the sun.
Pressure on top of head; better pressure.
Sleeps into headache; dreads to sleep as she wakes with such a distressing headache.
Headaches from suppressed discharges.

Menopause: Fainting; flushing; flooding; headaches; depression; weakness.

Menses (Periods): Acrid, black, clotted, scanty, of short duration.
Suppressed.
Feels better as soon as menses starts.

Metrorrhagia (Bleeding from Uterus): Bleeding from uterus at menopause; blood fluid, thin.

Ovaries: Pain in left ovary – left extending to right.
Pain better from flow of blood.
Pain burning; pressing; sore and tender.
Stitching in left ovary.
Pain after labour.

Pregnancy: Aversion to company during.

Pre-Menstrual Tension: Stomach disturbance; nervous restless-ness; headaches.

Sexual Desire: Increased.

Sleeplessness: All symptoms are worse after sleep; afraid to go to sleep.
Sleeps into aggravation.
Wakens at night and cannot get to sleep again.
From anxiety.
Wakes in a fright.
She feels worse after sleep.
Cannot bear bedclothes to touch throat.

Uterus: Congestion before and during periods.
Displacement.
Inflammation.
Pain better flow of blood.
Sore and tenderness.

Varicose Ulcer: With bluish, purplish appearance.

Varicose Veins: With ulceration.

LILIUM TIGRINUM

Characteristics:

Profound depression; fears some organic and incurable disease.
Aimless.
Worse: Warm room.
Better: Fresh air.

Depression: Full of rush and torment.
Depressed.
Weepy.
Indifferent.
Fears sanity.
Frantic hurry.
Walks fast.

Leucorrhoea: Brown.

Menses (Periods): Cease when lying.

Ovaries: Pain bearing down whilst standing.
Pain lancinating; sharp; stinging.
Sore and tender.

Pre-Menstrual Tension: Irritability.

Uterus: Pain bearing down as if everything would fall out.
Bearing down pain better by crossing legs.
Bearing down pain during periods.
Displacement.
Prolapse.

Vagina: Itching.

Vulva: Bearing down pain pressing on vulva.

LYCOPODIUM

Characteristics:

Intellectually keen but physically weak.
Upper part of body thin, lower part dropsical.
Very apprehensive – anticipation – before delivering address, lecture etc, but fine as soon as she gets going.
Likes to be alone but somebody in the next room or other part of the house.
Weeps when thanked.
Good appetite but a few mouthfuls fills up and she feels bloated.
Excessive accumulation of wind in lower abdomen.
Fullness – flatulence – distension.
Intolerance of tight clothing.
Symptoms begin on right side and often move to the left.
Red sand in urine.
Craves sweets.
Worse: 4 to 8 pm (no other remedy has this as such an outstanding symptom).
Worse: Cold food and drink; oysters; warm room.
Better: Warm food and drink (and much prefers it); open air; movement.

Breasts: Mastitis.
Nipples burning; cracked.
Sore fissures, covered with scurf.
Bleeding from ducts.

Constipation: No desire for days yet rectum full.
No urging.
Stool hard, difficult, small.
After stool feeling as if much remained – unpassed.
Spasmodic constriction of anus preventing stool.
Much flatus.

Cystitis: Turbid, milky urine with offensive sediment.
Heaviness of bladder.
Urging to urinate; must wait a long time for it to pass.
Constant bearing down sensation.
Copious red sand in urine.
Involuntary urination in sleep.
Passes enormous quantities of urine, very clear.

Depression: Melancholy, afraid to be alone.
Mind tired, forgetful, worried.
Distrustful, suspicious, fault-finding.

Diarrhoea: Stools pale, putrid, thin, brown, mixed with hard lumps. Thin, yellow or reddish-yellow fluid.

Headaches: Pressing pain on top of head worse 4 to 8 pm and from lying down or stooping.
Throbbing pain after coughing.
Pain over eyes with severe cold.
Pain in temples as if they were screwed together.
Tearing pains in back of head, better fresh air.

Leucorrhoea: Acrid and excoriating.
Gushing with burning in vagina.

Menses (Periods): Absent.
Late, protracted, suppressed.
Too profuse.

Ovaries: Enlarged.
Inflammation.
Pain in right ovary – from right to left.
Boring pain.

Pre-Menstrual Tension: Irritable, depressed.
Tummy disturbance.

Sexual Intercourse: Painful.

Uterus: Inflammation.
Polypus.

Vagina: Itching, burning, dry.

Varicose Ulcer: With burning pain, worse at night.

Varicose Veins: During pregnancy; painful.

MERCURIUS SOLUBILIS

Characteristics:

Trembling.
Weakness.
Sweat.
Profuse perspiration which does not relieve.
Salivation with intense thirst.
Mouth offensive – tongue large, flabby, shows imprint of teeth.
Worse: Night; warmth of bed.

Anxiety and Fear: Anxiety and apprehension.
Fearful dreams.
Hasty, hurried, restless, anxious, impulsive.

Breasts: Swelling.
Sore.
Painful and full of milk during periods.
Mastitis.
Nipples cracked.

Depression: Impulse to kill or commit suicide.
As though some evil is impending.
Worse at night with sweat.

Diarrhoea: Stools, slimy, even bloody, undigested, pitch-like, tenacious; yellow, dark, green, mucous and bloody.
Sour, excoriating anus.
Clay-coloured, slimy, offensive stools preceded by anxiety, trembling, faintness followed by chilliness.

Headaches: Tension about scalp as if bandaged.
One sided tearing pains.
Catarrhal headaches.
Much heat in head.

Leucorrhoea: Worse at night.
Acrid, excoriating, greenish and bloody.
Sensation of rawness in parts.

Miscarriage: Around the third month.

Ovaries: Inflammation.
Stinging pains.

Pregnancy: Morning sickness with profuse salivation.

Sleeplessness: On account of anxiety.
From itching and from seeing frightful faces.
Frequent waking.
Awake until around 3 am.
Night sweats.

Vagina: Inflammation.

Varicose Ulcer: Worse warmth.

NATRUM MURIATICUM

Characteristics:

Ill effects of grief, fright, anger.
Consolation aggravates; wants to be alone to cry.
Depressed; moody.
Very irritable.
Great weakness and weariness.
All mucous membranes dry.
Craves salt.
Very thirsty.
Worse: Noise; music; warm room; consolation; sea-shore (can be better sea-shore); heat and cold.
Better: Open air; cold bathing.

Constipation: Stool hard, difficult, crumbling.
Anus torn, bleeding, smarting, burning after stool.
Passes blood with stool.
Worse at periods.

Depression: Before periods; during pregnancy.
Very moody.

Diarrhoea: Chronic, watery; with fever, dry mouth, thirst.
Worse movement; much fetid flatus.
Green, bloody, watery or brownish.
Stools mostly during day.
Involuntary stools.

Headaches: Blinding headaches; throbbing; feels as if lots of little hammers were knocking on the brain.
Worse in morning on waking, after a period from sunrise to sunset.
Chronic headaches, congestive with nausea and vomiting.

Leucorrhoea: Albuminous; greenish, like boiled starch.
White, transparent, acrid, watery.

Menses (Periods): Copious, thin, frequent, late; pale, protracted, scanty, irregular.
First period in girls delayed.
Suppressed.

Pregnancy: Involuntary urination, vertigo, depression.

Pre-Menstrual Tension: With depression and headaches.

Sexual Intercourse: Aversion to.

Sterility: If other symptoms agree this remedy will help.

Uterus: Displacement of.
Prolapse, worse morning.
Pain bearing down, worse morning.
Labour pains weak.

Vagina: Dryness; painful intercourse.
Itching.

Varicose Veins: In legs.

NITRIC ACID

Characteristics:

Irritability.
Pains as from splinters.
Sticking pains.
Worse: Cold climate and also in hot weather.

Breasts: Nipples cracked; very sensitive.
Sticking pains like splinters.
Discoloured.

Constipation: Desire but little passes. Feels as if stool stayed in rectum and could not be expelled.
Ineffectual urging.
Colic.
Stools hard, preceded by great pressure followed by mucous discharge.
Straining without stool.
Burning in rectum.

Depression: Before periods.
Hopeless despair; anxious about illness; mind weak and wandering.
Nervous; fits of rage and despair.

Diarrhoea: Bloody stools; mucus putrid; yellow-white fluid.
Loose mornings.
Green, slimy, acrid diarrhoea.

Haemorrhoids: Chronic, pendulous, pain when touched.
Slimy, bleeding after every stool.
Worse warm weather.

Headaches: Sensation of band round head.
Headache from pressure of hat.
Fullness of head; worse noise.
Scalp sensitive.

Leucorrhoea: After periods, worse walking.
Acrid, excoriating; bloody, brown, greenish, offensive; thin, watery.
Ropy, stringy, tenacious.
Causes itching.

Menopause: With flooding.

Menses (Periods): Early, profuse; like muddy water.
With pain in back, hips and thighs.

Metrorrhagia (Bleeding from Uterus): Bleeding between periods after childbirth; fluid.

Pre-Menstrual Tension: Nervous restlessness and depression.

Uterus: Burning pain.
Haemorrhage from.

Vagina: Inflammation of.
Pain burning, stitching.
Itching after intercourse.

Varicose Ulcer: With burning pain, worse at night.

NUX MOSCHATA

Characteristics:

Complaints cause sleepiness.
Tendency to fainting fits.
Changeable moods – laughing and crying.
Extreme dryness of mucous membranes.
Worse: Cold.
Better: Warmth.

Menopause: With fainting.

Menses (Periods): Copious, too early, too frequent, too soon.
Irregular, late, dark, thick.
Variableness of periods; irregularity of time and quantity.
Feels better for periods.

Miscarriage: Tendency to.

Pregnancy: Vomiting with intense sleepiness and faintness.
Confusion of mind from mental exertion.

NUX VOMICA

Characteristics:

Very irritable, fiery temperament, impatient.
Can get excited, angry, spiteful and malicious.
Very particular and careful people.
Easily offended; anxious; depressed.
Sullen; fault-finding.
Over-sensitive to noise, slightest noise; strong odours; bright light; music. Feels everything too strongly.
Quick in movement.
Very chilly and when unwell in spite of layers of clothing and hugging the fire, still feels cold.
Worse: Cold; dry winds; east winds; morning; over-eating; over-drinking.
Better: Warm, wet weather; evening; after a nap.

Anxiety and Fear: Anxiety with irritability.
Great anxiety of mind with no particular cause.
Easily frightened.
Fears to be alone.

Constipation: Frequent and ineffectual desire or passing small quantities at each attempt.
Feeling as if part remained unexpelled.
Alternate constipation and diarrhoea.

Haemorrhoids: Itching, blind, very painful after ineffectual urging.
Burning, smarting and sticking.
Pains in rectum some hours after stool.

Headaches: Congestive; connected with gastric, abdominal or haemorrhoidal troubles.
As if a nail driven through brain.
Stitching pains with nausea and sour vomiting.
On waking; after eating; on moving eyes.
Better wrapping up head; lying; warmth.

Leucorrhoea: Offensive.

Menopause: With flushing.

Menses (Periods): Too early; very irregular.
Copious, dark, frequent, protracted.
Pain during periods in sacrum and constant urging to stool.
Feels better during periods.

Metrorrhagia (Bleeding from Uterus): Bleeding from uterus between periods.

Pregnancy: Vomiting with great irritability, retching and constipation.
With frequent urging to stool and urination.

Pre-Menstrual Tension: Headache, hysteria, giddy feeling, tummy upsets, irritability.

Sexual Desire: Increased.

Sleeplessness: After mental strain; abuse of coffee, wine, alcohol or tobacco.
From too much study at night.
Wakes at 3 to 4 am when mind is full of ideas, then sleeps lightly from which she finds difficulty in waking. Tired on waking.
All complaints worse from morning sleep.

Uterus: Pain during periods.
Bearing down pain with urging at stool.
Cramping pain compelling her to double up.
Cramping pains during menses.
Labour pains causing fainting.
Labour pains causing urging to stool.
Prolapse.

PHOSPHORUS

Characteristics:

Extremely sensitive.
Fearful of thunderstorms; being alone; of the dark; disease; death.
Very affectionate; they need it and give it, yet there can be an indifference.
Desire to be rubbed.
Much weakness and trembling.
Burning pains.
Haemorrhages bright and freely flowing.
Thirst for cold drinks which are vomited as soon as they become warm.
Worse: Physical or mental exertion; twilight; warm food or drink; from getting wet in hot weather; change of weather; evening; lying on painful side.
Better: Heat (everywhere except in stomach and head).
Dr Margaret Tyler says: 'Phosphorus complaints are worse from cold and cold weather, better from heat and warm applications, except for the complaints of head and stomach, which are ameliorated from cold'.

Anxiety and Fear: In pregnancy.
Very sensitive to external impressions.
Fearful of dark; thunder; that something will happen.
Anxious, filled with gloomy forebodings.
Fear and dread in the evening.
Uncommon fearfulness with great fatigue.

Breasts: Swelling, stitching pain.
Suppuration with burning, watery, offensive discharge.
Mastitis.
Nipples cracked and sore.

Constipation: Stools slender, long, dry, tough and hard like a dog's, voided with difficulty.
Very fetid, with flatus.

Diarrhoea: Painless, copious, debilitating, worse morning.
Stools profuse, watery, pouring away as if from a hydrant.
Light coloured, greenish or bloody.
Chronic painless diarrhoea.
Undigested food with much thirst for water during night.
Great weakness after stool.

Haemorrhoids: Bleeding.

Headaches: Chronic, congestive and throbbing.
Violent, with hunger or preceded by hunger.
Periodic headache from mental exertion.
Pains darting, tearing, shooting.
Worse noise, light and heat.

Leucorrhoea: Acrid, excoriating, profuse, smarting, instead of periods.

Menopause: With flushes of heat.

Menses (Periods): Bright red, copious, frequent, scanty, last too long.
Absence of periods.

Metrorrhagia (Bleeding from Uterus): Bleeding between periods when active.
Bright red, from fibroids, fluid, gushing, intermittent flow, profuse.

Ovaries: Inflammation.
Pain stitching.

Pregnancy: Sickness and vomiting associated with intense thirst for long cold drinks which are brought up again after five or ten minutes.

Pre-Menstrual Tension: Depressed, weepy.

Sexual Desire: Increased.

Sleeplessness: Sleepy during day, restless at night.
Wakened by vivid dreams.
Sleeplessness before midnight.
Drowsiness.
After excitement at theatre.

Uterus: Polypus.
Fibroids.

PLATINUM

Characteristics:

> Feels tall – mentally has great pride, looks down on others.
> Contempt for other people.
> Arrogant; proud; haughty.
> Numbness and coldness.
> Any disturbance of pride brings on symptoms.

Constipation: Difficult stools; sticky; adheres to rectum, like soft clay.
Frequent urging with inability to strain.
Chronic constipation.
Also of travellers who are constantly changing food and water.

Depression: Great anxiety; great dread of death which she thinks is near.
Mental disturbance after fright, grief or vexation.
Melancholy.

Menses (Periods): Clotted, copious, dark, frequent, protracted.
Mental troubles associated with suppressed periods.

Metrorrhagia (Bleeding from Uterus): Bleeding from uterus between periods.
Black.

Ovaries: Sensitive, burning.
Inflammation of ovaries with sterility.

Pre-Menstrual Tension: Hysterical.

Sexual Desire: Increased.

Uterus: Pain paroxysmal, sore, tender.
Bearing down pain.
Prolapse.
Polypus.

Vagina: Sensitive.

Vulva: Itching, voluptuous.

PODOPHYLLUM

Characteristics:

Suited to persons of bilious temperament.
Loquacity.
Depression.
Worse in hot weather.

Constipation: Clay-coloured, hard, dry and difficult stools.
Constipation alternating with diarrhoea.

Diarrhoea: Stools frequent, painless, watery, gushing out; yellow with sediment.
Green, sour with flatulence.
Chalk-like, undigested stools.
Muco-gelatinous stools preceded by griping colic.
Stools coated with shreds of yellow mucus.

Haemorrhoids: During pregnancy.

Headaches: Dull pressure, worse morning with hot face and bitter taste.
Rolling head from side to side with vomiting.

Menses (Periods): Suppressed.

Ovaries: Inflammation.
Pain in right ovary.

Uterus: Pain in uterus and right ovary with noises along ascending colon.
Prolapse from overlifting or over-straining during pregnancy.

PULSATILLA

Characteristics:

The temperament is mild and gentle but anger can appear, and irritability.

Tears come very easily; inclined to silent grief.

Conscientious, hates to be hussled.

Loves sympathy and fuss.

Changeable in everything; in disposition (like an April shower and sunshine); pains wander from joint to joint; no two stools are alike, etc.

Pulsatilla feels the heat; they must have air, it makes them feel much better.

Cannot eat fat, rich food, it makes them feel sick.

Thirstless, even with a fever.

Worse: Warm room, warm applications. Cannot bear heat in any form.

Better: Cool open air; walking slowly in open air but pains of Pulsatilla are accompanied by chilliness.

Anxiety and Fear: In pregnancy.

Forebodings; anxiety. Afraid of everybody.

Fright followed by diarrhoea.

Anxiety worse during rest, sitting and better by motion.

Breasts: Swelling.

Lactation, mild tearful women who have little milk.

Weeps every time child is fed.

Milk thin and watery; acrid milk.

Suppression of milk.

After weaning breasts swell, feel stretched and are intensely sore.

Milk continues to be secreted.

Mastitis.

Nipples burning, cracked.

Weeps whenever she nurses.

Constipation: Obstinate; stools hard and large.
Desire for stool, insufficient or no evacuation but instead yellowish, sometimes blood mixed with mucus.

Cystitis: Extremely painful, bloody, burning, smarting urine.
Dribbling urine on slightest provocation – coughing, sneezing, surprise, etc.
Great urgency – cannot delay.
Cannot lie on back without desire to urinate.
Involuntary urination in sleep, and during pregnancy.

Diarrhoea: Stools watery, usually at night; greenish-yellow, slimy, very changeable; like bile following rumbling in abdomen.
Offensive, corrosive; white and bloody mucus.

Haemorrhoids: Painful, protruding with smarting and soreness.
Generally with bleeding.

Headaches: Wandering stitches about head; pains extend to face and teeth; frontal pains.
Neuralgic pains commencing in right temple.
Headache from overwork.
Pressure on top of head.

Leucorrhoea: Acrid, excoriating, burning, cream-like.
While lying, milky, thin, watery.

Menses (Periods): First menses delayed in girls.
Absent or daytime only.
Changeable in appearance, clotted, dark, black, thick.
Intermittent, late, of short duration, protracted, scanty.
Suppressed or painful from getting feet wet.

Metrorrhagia (Bleeding from Uterus): Paroxysms of bleeding from uterus in between periods.

Miscarriage: Threatened; flow ceases and then returns in force, then ceases again, and so on.

Pre-Menstrual Tension: Nervous, restless, depressed; feeling of weakness.
Hysterical; headache; stomach disturbance.

Sexual Desire: Increased.

Sleeplessness: A fixed idea prevents sleep before midnight.
Wide awake evenings; does not want to go to bed; sound asleep when its time to get up.
Sleepless after eating too much too late.
Weeps because she cannot sleep.
Sleepless on account of great fear.

Subinvolution: If other symptoms agree this remedy will help.

Uterus: Congestion during periods; inflammation.
Pain before and during periods.
Pain paroxysmal, wandering, compels her to cry out.
Pain bearing down during period.
Pain cutting, griping, labour-like.
Pain labour – false, ineffectual, irregular, spasmodic, weak, ceasing.
After pains.
Sore, tenderness during intercourse.
Prolapse – during periods.

Varicose Ulcer: Bleeds easily; burning, painful. Worse warmth.

Varicose Veins: Painful, stinging; during pregnancy.

Vagina: Polypus.

SABINA

Characteristics:

Music is intolerable – produces nervousness.
Has a special action of the uterus.
Violent pulsations.
Worse: Least motion.
Better: In cool, fresh air.

Leucorrhoea: Like boiled starch; ropy, stringy, tenacious.

Menses (Periods): Copious, too early, too frequent, too soon.
Offensive, protracted, clotted.
Absent.

Metrorrhagia (Bleeding from Uterus): Bleeding from uterus between periods.
When active.
During and after labour.
Paroxysms – thin fluid.

Miscarriage: Tendency to, especially at the third month.

Ovaries: Inflammation after miscarriage.

Pregnancy: After pains intense.

Sexual desire: Increased.

Subinvolution: If other symptoms agree this remedy will help.

Uterus: Pain paroxysmal; bearing down; extends into thighs.
Pain cramping, paroxysmal.
Inflammation after miscarriage.
After pains.

SECALE CORNUTUM

Characteristics:

Debility, anxiety though appetite and thirst may be excessive.
All conditions better from cold, even coldness better cold!

Diarrhoea: Olive green, thin, putrid, bloody stools with icy coldness and intolerance of being covered, with great exhaustion.
Involuntary stools, no sensation of passing.

Leucorrhoea: Brownish, offensive.

Menses (Periods): Colic with coldness and intolerance of heat.
Irregular, copious, dark.

Metrorrhagia (Bleeding from Uterus): Continuous oozing of watery blood until next period.

Miscarriage: Threatened about the third month.

Pregnancy: During labour no expulsion though everything is relaxed.
After pains.

Sleeplessness: Of drug and liquor habitues.

SEPIA

Characteristics:

Great indifference to family (to husband and often children) and friends.
Averse to work; loses interest in what she ordinarily loves.
Irritable.
Easily offended.
Anxious.
Dreads to be alone.
Nervous, jumpy, hysterical.
Weeps when telling symptoms.
Depressed. Hates sympathy and weeps if it is offered.
Wants to get away to be quiet.
Weakness; weariness.
Pains travel upwards.
A 'ball' sensation in inner parts.
Faints when kneeling.
Feels the cold, must have air.
Gnawing hunger.
Craves vinegar and sour things; aversion to meat, fat, often bread and milk.
Worse: Damp; left side; after sweating; cold; cold air; east winds; sultry, moist weather.
Better: Exercise; pressure; warmth of bed; hot applications.

Anxiety and Fear: Fearfulness, cannot be alone for a minute.
Very fearful and frightened.
Fear of real and imaginary things.
Anxious dreams.

Breasts: Nipples, deep, sore cracks across crown of nipple.

Constipation: Ineffectual urging, days with no urging, then an effort as if in labour.
Stools not hard, but with much straining.
Feeling as if a 'ball in rectum'.
Straining and sweating with stool.
Stool insufficient, retarded like sheep's dung.
Pain in rectum long after stool.

Cystitis: Must keep her mind on neck of bladder or she will pass urine.

Depression: Before periods.
Despair about her miserable life; resigned despair.
Aversion to occupation and complete indifference to family.
Depressed about health and domestic affairs.
Absence of all joy.

Diarrhoea: Jelly-like stools with colic; green mucus, sour smelling, debilitating.

Headaches: Nervous, bilious, periodic, violent.
Better lying quiet and often cured by sleep.
Better, too, sometimes from violent motion.
Worse stooping, jarring, coughing, light.
Better hard exercise, tight bandage or applied heat.
Headaches at back of head with nausea and vomiting.
Better for sleep.

Leucorrhoea: Acrid, excoriating, albuminous, bloody, burning, copious.
Greenish, gushing before and between periods.
Milky, offensive in pregnancy.
Transparent, white, yellow with much itching.
Worse: mornings.

Menopause: With anxiety: fainting, flooding, flushing; headache and weakness.

Menses (Periods): Absent.
Late, scanty, one day only.
Early, profuse.
Bearing down pain.

Metrorrhagia (Bleeding from Uterus): Bleeding from uterus in between periods at menopause.

Miscarriage: Tendency to, especially around 5th to 7th month.

Pregnancy: Involuntary urination.

Pre-Menstrual Tension: With depression; nervous restlessness; headaches and stomach upsets.
Intense nausea and morning sickness aggravated by odour.

Sexual Intercourse: Aversion to; enjoyment absent.

Sleeplessness: Wakens at around 3 am, and cannot go to sleep again.
Frequent waking from sleep without cause.
Sleeplessness from thoughts rushing into the mind.
Restless sleep.

Sterility: If other symptoms agree this remedy will help.

Subinvolution: If other symptoms agree this remedy will help.

Uterus: Displacement, prolapse, congestion, heaviness.
Enlarged.
Pains, bearing down, morning and afternoon.
Pains, bearing down as if everything would drop out, better crossing legs.
Pains, bearing down during periods.
Pains, griping, labour-like, excessive, distressing.
Pains, sore and tenderness before periods.
Pains, stitching.
Polypus.

Vagina: Dryness.
Inflammation of.
Itching from leucorrhoea, during pregnancy.
Pain after intercourse.
Prolapse.

Vulva: Pain, pressing on, worse standing.
Pain worse urging to urinate.

SILICA

Characteristics:

Want of grit – moral and physical.
Yielding, faint-hearted, anxious.
Very sensitive to all impressions.
Easily irritated over trifles; touchy and self-willed.
Fixed ideas.
Intolerance of alcohol.
Suppurative processes.
Under nourished from imperfect assimilation.
Feels the cold.
Worse: Morning; uncovering; damp.
Better: Warmth; wrapping up head; in the summer; in wet or humid weather.

Anxiety and Fear: Dreads to appear in public.
Nervous exhaustion from brain-fag.
Dread of failure.
Retiring, wants to shirk everything.
'Anything for a quiet life.'
Dreads undertaking anything.

Breasts: Inflamed, swollen, hard, sensitive whilst nursing.
Lactation; sharp pains in breast or uterus; pain in back.
Pure blood flows every time child is put to breast.
Aversion to mother's milk.
Vomits after nursing.
Milk suppressed.
Inflamed breast, deep red in centre, swollen, hard, sensitive, constant.
Burning prevents rest.
Mastitis.
Nipples burning, cracked, sore, inflamed, nipple drawn in like a tunnel.

Constipation: Stool large or composed of hard lumps, light coloured; expulsions difficult from inactivity of rectum.
When partly expelled it slips back.
Always constipated before and during period.

Diarrhoea: Stools pap-like, offensive, contain undigested food.
Painless but with great exhaustion.

Haemorrhoids: Very painful; protrude during stool.

Headaches: Chronic sick headache with nausea and sometimes vomiting.
Begins in nape of neck and works over top of head to eyes, often the right is worse.
Better: Pressure; wrapping up head warmly; applied heat.

Leucorrhoea: Acrid during urination; excoriating, copious, gushing, milky.

Menses (Periods): Acrid; late; suppressed; absent.

Ovaries: Pains sharp while nursing.

Uterus: Pain while nursing child.
After pains when child nurses.
Polypus.

Vagina: Itching, very sensitive.

Varicose Ulcer: Burning, worse at night.

Vulva: Itching, very sensitive.

SULPHUR

Characteristics:

This remedy is known as the ragged philosopher.
Selfish, lazy and untidy people who often fling themselves into a chair with one leg draped over an arm. They are philosophical, wanting to know the 'Why's and wherefore's'.
Skin burning with itching, worse from warmth of bed.
Red orifices; eyes, nose, ears, lips and anus.
Sinking feeling mid-morning.
Worse standing.
Discharges offensive; acrid and excoriating, making part over which they flow red and burning.
Dislike of water; of washing.
Cat-nap sleep.
Worse: Warmth of bed; morning.
Better: Dry, warm weather.

Anxiety and Fear: Great anxiety in bed at full moon.
Fear for others.
Fear that she would take cold in open air.
Anxious dreams.

Breasts: After nursing nipples smart and burn; sore.
Breasts look unwashed.
Mastitis.
Nipples chap badly.
Nipples cracked.

Constipation: Frequent unsuccessful desire for stool.
A feeling as though something is left behind after stool.
Stool hard as if burnt.
Every 2, 3 or 4 days, hard and difficult.
Stool large, painful, held back because of pain.
Alternation of constipation and diarrhoea.

Diarrhoea: At night with colic; watery, white stools, smelling sour.
Driving out of bed in morning, painless.
Watery, involuntary as if bowels too weak to retain contents.

Haemorrhoids: Blind or flowing dark blood with violent bearing down pains from small of back towards anus.
Pulsating in anus all day.
Itching, burning and stinging in anus.
Anus swollen.
Stools excoriate.

Headaches: Burning on top of head (also in hands and soles of feet).
Heaviness of head; worse stooping, moving, sitting and lying.
Headaches from pressure of hat, better head uncovered.
Periodic, sick headache with nausea and vomiting.
Often this occurs every 7 days.
Worse movement, eating and drinking.

Leucorrhoea: Burning, excoriating, yellow.

Menopause: With fainting and flushing.

Menses (Periods): Late, scanty, of short duration.
Thick, black, acrid making parts sore.

Metrorrhagia (Bleeding from Uterus): Bleeding from uterus during menopause.

Miscarriage: Tendency to.

Pregnancy: Vomiting and sickness but patient is cheerful and hungry in spite of it.

Pre-Menstrual Tension: Headaches; stomach disturbance.

Sleeplessness: Very drowsy during the day but wakeful at night.
Tosses around, nervous.
Great flow of thoughts prevent sleep and cause perspiration.
Wakes at 3, 4 or 5 am, and cannot sleep again.
Best and soundest sleep late mornings.
Soles burn at night, puts feet out of bed.
Worse warmth of bed.

Subinvolution: If other symptoms agree this remedy will help.

Uterus: Pains bearing down at night in bed.

Vagina: Pains burning; itching.
Inflammation of.

REPERTORY

Anxiety and Fear: Acon; Arn; Ars; Bell; Bor; Bry; Calc; Cim; Gels; Graph; Kali C; Lach; Merc; Nux V; Phos; Puls; Sep; Sil; Sul.

Breasts: Bell; Bry; Cham; Con; Graph; Lach; Sil.

Constipation: Alum; Apis; Bry; Calc; Caust; Cocc; Con; Graph; Lyc; Nat M; Nit Ac; Nux V; Phos; Plat; Pod; Puls; Sep; Sil; Sul.

Cystitis: Arn; Apis; Bell; Caust; Cham; Lach; Lyc; Puls.

Depression: Apis; Ars; China; Cim; Lil T; Lyc; Merc; Nat M; Nit Ac; Plat; Sep.

Diarrhoea: Alum; Apis; Ars; Bry; Calc; Cham; China; Ip; Lach; Lyc; Merc; Nat M; Nit Ac; Phos; Pod; Puls; Sec; Sep; Sil; Sul.

Haemorrhoids: Alum; Apis; Ars; Calc; Caust; Graph; Lach; Nit Ac; Nux V; Phos; Pod; Puls; Sil; Sul.

Headaches: Acon; Arn; Apis; Ars; Bell; Bry; Calc; China; Cocc; Gels; Lach; Lyc; Merc; Nat M; Nit Ac; Nux V; Phos; Pod; Puls; Sep; Sil; Sul.

Lactation: Bell; Puls; Sil.

Leucorrhoea: Acon; Alum; Ars; Bor; Calc; Caul; Caust; Cham; Cocc; Graph; Kali C; Kreos; Lil T; Lyc; Merc; Nat M; Nit Ac; Nux V; Phos; Puls; Sab; Sec; Sep; Sil; Sul.

Mastitis: Arn; Apis; Bry; Cham; Con; Lach; Lyc; Merc; Phos; Puls; Sil; Sul.

Menopause: Acon; Bell; Bor; Calc; Cim; Graph; Kali C; Lach; Nit Ac; Nux M; Nux V; Phos; Sep; Sul.

Menses (Periods): Acon; Alum; Apis; Ars; Bell; Bor; Bry; Calc; Caul; Caust; Cham; China; Cim; Cocc; Con; Gels; Graph; Ip; Kali C; Kreos; Lach; Lil T; Lyc; Nat M; Nit Ac; Nux M; Nux V; Phos; Plat; Pod; Puls; Sab; Sec; Sep; Sil; Sul.

Metrorrhagia (Bleeding from Uterus): Bell; Calc; Cham; China; Ip; Kreos; Lach; Nit Ac; Nux V; Phos; Plat; Puls; Sab; Sec; Sep; Sul.

Miscarriage: Acon; Arn; Apis; Bell; Calc; Caul; Cham; Cim; Gels; Kali C; Merc; Nux M; Puls; Sab; Sec; Sep; Sul.

Nipples: Arn; Ars; Caust; Cham; Con; Graph; Lyc; Merc; Nit Ac; Phos; Puls; Sep; Sil; Sul.

Ovaries: Acon; Apis; Ars; Bell; Bry; China; Con; Graph; Lach; Lil T; Lyc; Merc; Phos; Plat; Pod; Sab; Sil.

Pregnancy: Acon; Arn; Ars; Caust; Cim; Gels; Ip; Kreos; Lach; Merc; Nat M; Nux M; Nux V; Phos; Sab; Sec; Sep; Sul.

Pre-Menstrual Tension: Acon; Alum; Bry; Calc; Caul; Cham; Cim; Cocc; Con; Gels; Graph; Kali C; Kreos; Lach; Lil T; Lyc; Nat M; Nit Ac; Nux V; Phos; Plat; Puls; Sep; Sul.

Sexual Desire Diminished: Caust.

Sexual Desire Increased: Calc; Con; Lach; Nux V; Phos; Plat; Puls; Sab.

Sexual Intercourse: Graph; Nat M; Sep.

Sleeplessness: Acon; Arn; Ars; Bell; Bry; Calc; Cham; Cocc; Kali C; Lach; Merc; Nux V; Phos; Puls; Sec; Sep; Sul.

Sterility: Bor; Merc; Sep.

Subinvolution: Bell; Calc; Caul; Cim; Puls; Sab; Sep; Sul.

Uterus: Acon; Apis; Ars; Bell; Bry; Calc; Caul; Caust; Cham; Cim; Cocc; Con; Graph; Ip; Kali C; Kreos; Lach; Lil T; Lyc; Nat M; Nit Ac; Nux V; Phos; Plat; Pod; Puls; Sab; Sep; Sil; Sul.

Vagina: Acon; Alum; Bor; Calc; Caul; Caust; Con; Graph; Kali C; Kreos; Lil T; Lyc; Merc; Nat M; Nit Ac; Plat; Puls; Sep; Sil; Sul.

Varicose Veins: Arn; Ars; Calc; Caust; Graph; Kreos; Lach; Lyc; Nat M; Puls; Sul.

Varicose Ulcer: Arn; Ars; Calc; Graph; Kali C; Lach; Lyc; Merc; Nit Ac; Puls; Sil; Sul.

Vulva: Alum; Bor; Calc; Kreos; Lil T; Plat; Sep; Sil

CHARACTERISTICS

MENTAL

AFFECTIONATE: Phos.
AGITATION: Cim.
AIMLESS: Lil T.
ALONE, LIKES TO BE, BUT SOMEBODY IN NEXT ROOM: Lyc.
ANGER: Bell; Nux V.
ANGER, ILL EFFECTS OF: Nat M.
ANGUISH: Ars.
ANXIETY: Acon: Nux V; Sec; Sep; Sil.
ANXIETY IN STOMACH: Kali C.
APATHY REGARDING ILLNESS: Gels.
APPREHENSION: Calc: Caust; Lyc.
ARROGANT: Plat.
AVERSE TO WORK: Sep.

CHANGEABLE IN EVERYTHING: Puls.
CONTEMPT FOR OTHERS: Plat.
CONTRADICTION, CANNOT BEAR: Cocc.

DEBILITY: Sec.
DEBILITY FROM LOSS OF FLUIDS: China.
DEPRESSION: Caust; Cim; Lil T; Nat M; Nux V; Pod; Sep.
DESIRE TO BE RUBBED: Phos.
DIZZINESS: Con; Gels.
DREAD OF BEING ALONE: Sep.
DREAD OF DOWNWARD MOTION: Bor.
DROWSINESS: Gels.
DULLNESS: Gels.

EXCITED: Nux V.
EXHAUSTION: Ars.

FAINT-HEARTED: Sil.
FAINTING, TENDENCY TO: Nux V.
FAINTNESS: Calc.
FAINTNESS, SITTING UP IN BED: Bry.
FASTIDIOUS: Ars; Nux V.
FAULT-FINDING: Nux V.
FEAR OF BEING ALONE: Phos.
FEAR OF THE DARK: Phos.
FEAR OF DEATH: Acon; Phos.
FEAR OF DISEASE: Phos.
FEAR OF THE FUTURE: Acon.
FEAR OF THUNDER: Phos.
FEAR WITH VOMITING: Acon.
FEARFUL: Acon; Ars; Calc; Gels; Lil T.
FIERY TEMPER: Nux V.
FIXED IDEAS: Sil.
FORGETFUL: Kreos.
FRIGHT, ILL EFFECTS OF: Nat M.
FRIGHTENED: Acon; Ars; Bor.

GRIEF, ILL EFFECTS FROM: Nat M.

HASTY: Alum.
HOLLOWNESS, SENSATION OF: Cocc.
HURRIED: Alum.
HYSTERICAL: Sep.

IMPATIENT: Cham; Ip; Nux V.
INABILITY TO CONTROL TEMPER: Cham.
INDIFFERENCE: Sep.
INTELLECTUALLY KEEN BUT PHYSICALLY WEAK: Lyc.
INTOLERANCE OF ALCOHOL: Sil.
INTOLERANCE OF ANYTHING TIGHT: Lach; Lyc.
INTOLERANCE OF COLD WEATHER: Kali C.
INTOLERANCE OF LIGHT: Graph.
IRRITABILITY: Bry; Caust; Cham; Cocc; Ip; Kali C; Kreos; Nat M; Nit Ac; Nux V; Sep.

JEALOUS: Apis.
JEALOUS, INSANELY: Lach.

LAZY: Sul.
LOQUACITY: Pod.

MALICIOUS: Nux V.
MOODY: Nat M; Nux V.
MUSIC CAUSES PATIENT TO CRY: Graph.
MUSIC INTOLERABLE: Sab.

NERVOUS: Bor: Sep.
NIGHT-WATCHING, EFFECTS OF: Cocc.
NOISE, HYPER-SENSITIVE TO: Kali C.
NUMBNESS: Con.

OFFENDED EASILY: Nux V; Sep.

PAIN, HYPER-SENSITIVE TO: Kali C.
PARTICULAR, VERY: Nux V.
PEEVISH: Kreos.
PHILOSOPHICAL: Sul.
PRIDE, GREAT: Plat.
PROSTRATION: Ars.

RESTLESSNESS: Acon; Ars.

SADNESS: Cocc.
SCORNFUL: Ip.
SELFISH: Sul.
SELF-WILLED: Sil.
SENSITIVE: Sil.
SENSITIVE, OVER: Cham; Phos.
SENSITIVE TO LIGHT: Nux V.
SENSITIVE TO MUSIC: Nux V.
SENSITIVE TO NOISE: Kali C; Nux V.
SENSITIVE TO SUDDEN NOISE: Bor.
SENSITIVE TO STRONG ODOURS: Nux V.
SENSITIVE TO TOUCH: Kali C.
SLEEP, RESTLESS: Bell.
SLEEPINESS, COMPLAINTS FROM: Nux M.
SLOW: Calc.
SPITEFUL: Nux V.
STUPID: Kreos.

SULLEN: Nux V.
SUSPICIOUS: Apis; Lach.
SYMPATHETIC: Caust.
SYMPATHY, LOATHES: Sep.
SYMPATHY LOVES: Puls.

TEARFUL: Apis.
TEMPERAMENT BILIOUS: Pod.
TEMPERAMENT GENTLE: Puls.
TEMPERAMENT MILD: Puls.
TENSION: Acon.
THINKING, SLOWNESS IN: Cocc.
TIME PASSES TOO QUICKLY: Cocc.
TIME PASSES TOO SLOWLY: Alum.
TOUCHY: Sil.
TREMBLING: Con; Gels; Merc; Phos.

VEXATION, AILMENTS FROM: Ip.

WANT OF MENTAL GRIT: Sil.
WEARINESS: Nat M.
WEAKNESS: Merc; Phos; Sep.
WEAKNESS: PARALYTIC; MENTAL: Con.
WEEPS EASILY: Puls.
WEEPS WHEN TELLING SYMPTOMS: Sep.
WEEPS WHEN THANKED: Lyc.
WHINING: Apis, Cham.
WORRY: Ars.

YIELDING: Sil.

CHARACTERISTICS

PHYSICAL

AVERSION, MEAT ETC: Sep.
AWKWARD, DROPS THINGS: Apis.

BALL, SENSATION INNER PARTS: Sep.
BREATHLESS: Calc.

CATNAP SLEEP: Sul.
CAUSED BY DISTURBANCE OF PRIDE: Plat.
CAUSED BY EXPOSURE TO, COLD, DRY WINDS: Acon.
COLD ALWAYS, BUT CRAVES AIR: Graph.
COLD WITH NUMBNESS: Plat.
COMPLAINTS AFTER LOSS OF FLUIDS: China.
COMPLAINTS DEVELOP SLOWLY: Bry.
CONSTRICTED SENSATION: Apis.
CRAVES FRESH AIR: Puls.
CRAVES INDIGESTIBLE THINGS: Calc.
CRAVES SALT: Nat M.
CRAVES SOUR THINGS: Sep.
CRAVES SWEETS: Lyc.
CRAVES VINEGAR: Sep.
CRAVINGS ABNORMAL: Alum.

DISCHARGES, ACRID: Sul.
DISCHARGES, BURNING: Apis.
DISCHARGES, EXCORIATING: Kreos; Sul.
DISCHARGES, OFFENSIVE: Kreos; Sul.
DISTENTION, FEELING OF: Lyc.
DRYNESS OF MUCOUS MEMBRANES: Alum; Bry; Merc; Nat M;
Nux V.

ERUPTIONS STICKY: Graph.

FACE FLUSHED: Bell.
FAIR: Calc.
FAT: Calc.
FLABBY: Calc.
FLATULENCE: Lyc.
FLATULENCE IN LOWER ABDOMEN: Lyc.
FOOD, FEW MOUTHFULS FILL: Lyc.
FULLNESS, FEELING OF: Lyc.
FUNCTIONING SLUGGISH: Alum.

GLANDS, ENLARGEMENT OF: Calc.
GREATER THE FLOW, GREATER THE PAIN: Cim.

HAEMORRHAGE, BRIGHT RED: Ip.
HAEMORRHAGE, FREELY FLOWING: Phos.
HAEMORRHAGE, PROFUSE: China; Ip.
HAEMORRHAGE, PROFUSE WITH FAINTING: China.

INJURIES TRAUMATIC: Arn.

MOUTH OFFENSIVE: Merc.

NAUSEA PERSISTENT: Ip.
NAUSEA AND VOMITING WITH CLEAN TONGUE: Ip.

OBESITY: Graph.
OEDEMA: Apis.
ORIFICES, RED: Sul.

PAIN, BRUISED: Arn.
PAIN, BURNING: Apis; Ars; Bell; Caust; Phos.
PAIN, CUTTING: Kali C.
PAIN, RAWNESS: Caust.
PAIN, SHARP: Kali C.
PAIN, SORENESS: Caust.
PAIN, STICKING: Nit Ac.
PAIN, STINGING: Apis.
PAIN, STITCHING: Bry.
PAIN, TEARING: Bry.

PAIN, THROBBING: Bell.
PAINS AS FROM SPLINTERS: Nit Ac.
PAINS TRAVEL UPWARDS: Sep.
PARALYSIS OF SINGLE PARTS: Caust.
PROSTRATION, MUSCULAR: Gels.
PULSATIONS, VIOLENT: Sab.
PUPILS DILATED: Bell.

RESTLESSNESS: Acon; Ars; Cham.
RIGHT TO LEFT: Lyc.

SALIVATION WITH INTENSE THIRST: Merc.
SAND, RED IN URINE: Lyc.
SENSITIVE TO COLD AIR: Cocc.
SENSITIVE TO HOT AIR: Cocc.
SINKING FEELING, MORNING: Sul.
SKIN BURNING: Bell; Sul.
SKIN BURNING WITH ITCHING: Sul.
SKIN CRACKED: Graph.
SKIN DIRTY: Caust.
SKIN DRY: Bell.
SKIN ROUGH: Graph.
SKIN SALLOW: Caust.
SKIN WHITE: Caust.
SLEEPS INTO AGGRAVATION: Lach.
SORENESS: Arn.
SOUR STOOL: Calc.
SOUR URINE: Calc.
SUDDEN BEGINNING OF ACUTE ILLNESS: Acon.
SUPPURATIVE PROCESSES: Sil.
SWEAT COPIOUS DURING SLEEP: Con.
SWEAT EVEN IN COOL ROOM: Calc.
SWEAT PROFUSE, ESPECIALLY ON HEAD: Calc.
SWEAT SOUR, ESPECIALLY ON HEAD: Calc.
SWEAT WITHOUT THIRST: Apis.

TEMPERATURE, SUDDEN RISE: Bell.
THIRST FOR COLD DRINKS, VOMITED AS SOON AS WARM:
Phos.

THIRST FOR EXCESSIVE COPIOUS DRAUGHTS AT LONG INTERVALS: Bry.
THIRST FOR SMALL AMOUNTS FREQUENTLY: Ars.
THIRSTLESS: Apis.
THIRSTLESS EVEN WITH FEVER: Puls.
THIRSTY: Nat M.
TIREDNESS: Gels.
TONGUE FLABBY: Merc.
TONGUE LARGE: Merc.

UTERUS, WANT OF TONICITY: Caul.

WANT OF PHYSICAL GRIT: Sil.
WEAKNESS: Nat M.
WEAKNESS: PARALYTIC, PHYSICAL: Con.
WOMEN, CHILL: Graph.
WOMEN, CONSTIPATED: Graph.
WOMEN, OVER WEIGHT: Graph.
WRAPPED UP, MUST BE: Graph.

MODALITIES

BETTER

After breakfast: Calc.
Bending forward: Gels.
Cold applications: Apis.
Cold bathing: Nat M.
Cold room: Apis.
Cold things: Bry.
Constipated, when: Calc.
Dark, in: Graph.
Discharge, any: Lach.
Drawing up limbs: Calc.
Drink, warm: Lyc.
Evening: Nux V.
Exercise: Sep.
Hot applications: Sep.
Loosening garments: Calc.
Lying on back: Calc.
Lying on painful side: Bry.
Motion: Kreos.
Movement: Lyc.
Nap, after: Nux V.
Pressure: Bry; Sep.
Pressure; hard: China.
Rest: Bry.
Rubbing: Calc.
Summer: Sul.
Walking slowly: Puls.
Warm applications: Lach.
Warmth of bed: Sep.
Wrapping up: Graph.
Wrapping up head: Sil.

WEATHER BETTER

Air, cold: Apis.
Air, cool: Sab.
Air, fresh: Acon; Alum; China; Gels; Lil T; Nat M; Puls.
Air, open: Lyc; Puls.
Damp: Alum; Caust.
Dry: Calc; Sul.
Warm; Calc; Caust; China; Cim; Kreos; Nux M; Sul.
Warm, moist: Cham; Kali C; Nux V.
Warmth, except of head: Ars.
Warmth, except of head and stomach: Phos.
Wet or humid: Sil.

MODALITIES

WORSE

After midnight: Ars; Calc.
Around midnight: Acon.
Evening: Phos.
Morning: Sul.
Night: Ars; Merc.
On waking: Calc.
3 am: Kali C.
10 am: Gels.
4–8 pm: Lyc.

WEATHER WORSE

Air, cold: Ars, Calc, Sep.
Air, draught of: China.
Air, open: Calc; Kreos.
Change of weather: Phos.
Cold: Cim; Kreos; Nux M; Nux V; Sep.
Cold climate: Nit Ac.
Cold, damp: Arn.
Cold, wet: Calc.
Damp: Sep.
Heat: Apis; Bor; Bry; Cham; Graph; Nit Ac; Pod.
Heat and cold: Nat M.
Spring: Lach.
Sultry, moist: Sep.
Wet: Ars.
Wind, dry: Nux V.
Wind, dry, cold: Acon; Caust.
Wind, east: Nux V; Sep..

WORSE

Bad news: Gels.
Bathing: Calc.

Baths, hot: Apis.
Coffee: Kali C.
Cold applications: Ars.
Cold drinks: Ars; Lyc.
Cold food: Lyc.
Emotional upsets: Gels.
Excitement: Gels.
Exertion, mental and physical: Phos.
Food, rich and fat: Puls.
Hot drinks: Lach.
Left side: Lach.
Limbs, letting them hang down: Calc.
Lying: Kreos.
Lying on left side: Kali C.
Lying on painful side: Kali C; Phos.
Menses, after: Kreos.
Moon, full: Calc.
Moon, new: Calc.
Motion, least: Bry; Sab.
Music: Nat M.
Noise: Nat M.
Over drinking: Nux V.
Overeating: Nux V.
Oysters: Lyc.
Rest: Kreos.
Seashore: Nat M.
Side, left: Lach; Sep.
Sleep, after: Lach.
Standing: Sul.
Stooping: Calc.
Sweating, after: Sep.
Touch, slight: China, Kali C.
Twilight: Phos.
Warm applications: Puls.
Warm drink: Phos.
Warm food: Phos.
Warm room: Acon; Alum; Apis; Lil T; Lyc; Nat M; Puls.
Warmth at night: Graph.
Warmth of any kind: Puls.
Warmth of bed: Merc; Sul.
Wet, getting in warm weather: Phos.
Working in water: Calc.

REPERTORY OF EACH SECTION

Anxiety and Fear
ANXIETY ABOUT BUSINESS: Bry.
ANXIETY ABOUT THE FUTURE: Bry.
ANXIETY, ATTACKS OF: Arn.
ANXIETY, EXCESSIVE: Ars, Bell.
ANXIETY, GREAT, WITH NO PARTICULAR CAUSE: Nux V.
ANXIETY IN BED AT FULL MOON: Sul.
ANXIETY WHEN ALONE: Ars; Sep.
ANXIETY WITH IRRITABILITY: Nux V.
ANXIETY WITH IRRITABILITY AND RESTLESSNESS: Ars.
ANXIOUS DREAMS: Sep; Sil.
APPREHENSION: Graph; Merc.
APPREHENSION ABOUT THE FUTURE: Arn.
AVERSION TO BEING ALONE: Kali C.
DREADS TO APPEAR IN PUBLIC: Sil.
DREADS EVENING: Phos.
DREADS FAILURE: Sil.
DREADS UNDERTAKING ANYTHING NEW: Sil.
FEAR, AFTER LABOUR: Acon.
FEAR, BAD EFFECTS FROM: Gels.
FEAR OF BEING ALONE: Nux V.
FEAR OF BEING APPROACHED: Arn.
FEAR OF BEING POISONED: Lach.
FEAR OF DEATH: Ars; Lach.
FEAR OF DOWNWARD MOTION: Bor.
FEAR OF DYING IN CONFINEMENT: Acon.
FEAR OF EVENING: Phos.
FEAR OF EVERYBODY: Puls.
FEAR OF IMAGINARY THINGS: Bell; Calc; Sep.
FEAR OF HER DISEASE, SHE CANNOT RECOVER FROM IT: Kali C.
FEAR OF OTHERS: Sul.
FEAR OF THE DARK: Phos.

FEAR OF THE FUTURE: Calc.
FEAR OF THUNDER: Phos.
FEAR SHE WOULD TAKE COLD IN OPEN AIR: Sul.
FEARFUL: Sep.
FEARFUL DREAMS: Arn; Merc.
FEARFUL, EXTREMELY: Acon; Calc.
FEARFUL IF ANYTHING TOUCHES BODY LIGHTLY: Kali C.
FEARFUL IN PREGNANCY: Cim; Phos; Puls.
FIDGETY: Bor; Graph.
FOREBODINGS: Puls.
FOREBODINGS, GLOOMY: Phos.
FRIGHT, BAD EFFECTS FROM: Gels.
FRIGHT FOLLOWED BY DIARRHOEA: Puls.
FRIGHTENED: Sep.
HASTY: Merc.
HURRIED: Merc.
IMPULSIVE: Merc.
INDECISIVE: Graph.
LACKS COURAGE: Gels.
NERVOUS EXHAUSTION FROM BRAIN-FAG: Sil.
PALPITATION WITH GREAT ANXIETY: Acon; Calc.
RESTLESS: Merc.
RETIRING: Sil.
SENSITIVE TO EXTERNAL IMPRESSIONS: Phos.
SHOCKS FELT IN STOMACH: Kali C.
STARTLED EASILY: Bor.
STARTLED IN FRIGHT: Bell.
TIMID: Graph.
TREMORS, WANTS TO BE HELD: Gels.

BETTER MOTION: Puls.

WORSE DURING REST: Puls.
WORSE SITTING: Puls.
WORSE WAKING: Lach.

Breasts
BLOOD FLOWS WHEN CHILD IS PUT TO BREAST: Sil.
DISTENDED: Calc.
DRY: Bell.
ENLARGE BEFORE PERIODS: Con.

120

ENLARGE DURING PERIODS: Con.
HARDNESS: Graph; Sil.
HARDNESS, STONY: Bell.
INFLAMMATION: Bell; Sil.
LACTATION, AVERSION TO MOTHER'S MILK: Sil.
LACTATION, MILK CONTINUES TO BE SECRETED: Puls.
LACTATION, DISAGREEABLE, NAUSEATING TASTE: Calc.
LACTATION, DISAGREES: Calc.
LACTATION, EXCESSIVE WITH DEBILITY: Calc.
LACTATION, EXCESSIVE WITH FEVER: Calc.
LACTATION, EXCESSIVE WITH SWEAT: Calc.
LACTATION, FLOW TOO COPIOUS: Bell.
LACTATION, LITTLE, IN MILD, TEARFUL WOMEN: Puls.
LACTATION, PROFUSE SECRETION REFUSED BY CHILD: Calc.
LACTATION, SCANTY: Calc.
LACTATION, SUPPRESSED: Puls, Sil.
LACTATION, WATERY, THIN: Puls.
LAX: Con.
LOOK UNWASHED: Sul.
MASTITIS: Bell; Bry; Cham; Con; Lach; Lyc; Merc; Phos; Puls;
Sil; Sul.
MASTITIS, FROM INJURY: Arn.
NIPPLES, BLEEDING FROM DUCTS: Lyc.
NIPPLES, BLISTERED: Graph.
NIPPLES, CHAP BADLY: Sul.
NIPPLES, CRACKED: Ars; Caust; Cham; Graph; Lyc; Merc;
Nit Ac; Phos; Puls; Sil; Sul.
NIPPLES, CRACKS ACROSS CROWN: Sep.
NIPPLES, CRACKS DEEP: Sep.
NIPPLES, CRACKS SORE: Sep.
NIPPLES, DISCOLOURED: Nit Ac.
NIPPLES, DRAWN IN: Sil.
NIPPLES, INFLAMED: Cham; Sil.
NIPPLES, PAIN, BURNING: Ars; Con; Lyc; Puls; Sil.
NIPPLES, PAIN, BURNING AFTER NURSING: Sul.
NIPPLES, PAIN, SORE FISSURES COVERED WITH SCURF: Lyc.
NIPPLES, PAIN, SMARTING AFTER NURSING: Sul.
NIPPLES, PAIN, STICKING (LIKE SPLINTERS): Nit Ac.
NIPPLES, PAIN, STITCHING: Con.
NIPPLES, PAIN, TENDER: Cham.

NIPPLES, SENSITIVE: Nit Ac.
NIPPLES, SURROUNDED WITH HERPES: Caust.
PAIN, BURNING: Sil.
PAIN, SORE AFTER WEANING: Puls.
PAIN, SORE TENDER: Bry; Calc; Cham; Lach; Merc.
PAIN, STITCHING: Phos.
PAINFUL AND FULL OF MILK DURING PERIODS: Merc.
PAINFUL BEFORE PERIODS: Con.
PAINFUL DURING PERIODS: Bry; Con.
PAINFUL TO TOUCH: Con.
SENSITIVE WHILE NURSING: Sil.
SHRUNKEN: Con.
SWELLING, HOT: Calc.
SWOLLEN: Bry; Bell; Graph; Merc; Phos; Puls; Sil.
SWOLLEN AFTER WEANING: Puls.
SUPPURATION WITH BURNING: Phos.
SUPPURATION, OFFENSIVE: Phos.
SUPPURATION, WATERY: Phos.
VOMITS AFTER NURSING: Sil.
WEEPS EVERY TIME CHILD IS FED: Puls.
WITH SHARP PAINS IN BREAST ON NURSING: Sil.
WITH SHARP PAINS IN UTERUS ON NURSING: Sil.

Constipation
ALTERNATE CONSTIPATION AND DIARRHOEA: Nux V; Pod; Sul.
ANUS BLEEDING AFTER STOOL: Nat M.
ANUS BURNING AFTER STOOL: Nat M.
ANUS CONSTRICTION OF: Lyc.
ANUS SMARTING AFTER STOOL: Nat M.
ANUS TORN AFTER STOOL: Nat M.
BEFORE PERIOD: Sil.
CHRONIC: Plat.
CHRONIC OF TRAVELLERS: Plat.
CHRONIC WITH SEVERE HEADACHE: Bry.
COSTIVE: Lach.
DESIRE BUT LITTLE PASSES: Nit Ac.
DURING PERIOD: Sil.
FAINTS AFTER STOOL: Cocc.
FLATUS: Lyc.

FREQUENT UNSUCCESSFUL DESIRE: Sul.
INABILITY TO PASS STOOL: Cocc.
RECTUM BURNING: Nit Ac.
RECTUM BURNING AFTER STOOL: Bry; Con.
RECTUM, FEELING OF BALL IN: Sep.
RECTUM, FEELS AS IF PART REMAINS UNEXPELLED: Nux V; Sul.
RECTUM, INACTIVITY OF: Alum; Caust; Nit Ac; Sil.
RECTUM, PAINS LONG AFTER STOOL: Sep.
RECTUM, PARALYSED, SEEMS TO BE: Alum; Apis; Cocc.
STOOLS, ABSENT FOR DAYS: Apis; Lyc.
STOOLS, BLOOD WITH: Nat M.
STOOLS, CHALKY-WHITE: Calc.
STOOLS, CLAY-COLOURED: Calc; Pod.
STOOLS, CRUMBLING: Nat M.
STOOLS, DARK: Bry.
STOOLS, DIFFICULT: Lyc; Nat M; Sul.
STOOLS, DRY: Bry; Calc; Lyc; Nat M; Phos; Plat; Pod.
STOOLS, EVERY 2–3–4 DAYS: Sul.
STOOLS, FETID WITH FLATUS: Phos.
STOOLS, HARD: Alum; Bry; Calc; Con; Graph; Lyc; Nat M; Nit Ac; Phos; Pod; Puls.
STOOLS, HARD AS IF BURNT: Sul.
STOOLS, KNOTTY (LIKE SHEEP'S DUNG): Alum; Graph; Sep.
STOOLS, LARGE: Graph; Puls; Sil; Sul.
STOOLS, LONG: Phos.
STOOLS, OBSTINATE: Puls.
STOOLS, OFFENSIVE: Lach.
STOOLS, PAINFUL: Sul.
STOOLS, PASSED BETTER WHEN STANDING: Caust.
STOOLS, RETARDED: Sep.
STOOLS, SLENDER: Phos.
STOOLS, SMALL: Lyc.
STOOLS, SMELLING LIKE BAD EGGS: Calc.
STOOLS, SOFT (LIKE CLAY): Alum.
STOOLS, STICKY: Plat.
STOOLS, THIN: Lach.
STOOLS, TOUGH: Phos.
STOOLS, TREMBLING AND WEAKNESS AFTER: Con.
STOOLS, UNDIGESTED: Calc.

STOOLS, WHEN PARTLY EXPELLED SLIP BACK: Sil.
STRAINING AND SWEATING WITH STOOL: Sep.
STRAINING EVEN WITH SOFT STOOL: Alum.
STRAINING WITHOUT STOOL: Nit Ac.
STUBBORN: Calc.
URGE, NONE: Bry; Lyc.
URGE, NONE YET RECTUM FULL: Lyc.
URGING, FREQUENT WITH INABILITY TO STRAIN: Plat.
URGING, INEFFECTUAL EFFORTS: Caust; Con; Lach; Nit Ac; Nux V; Sep.
URGING, INEFFECTUAL WITH ANXIETY: Caust.
URGING, INEFFECTUAL WITH PAIN: Caust.
WITH COLIC: Nit Ac.
WITH PAIN IN BOWELS: Ars.
WITH SLIMY MUCUS: Graph.

BETTER WHEN CONSTIPATED: Calc.

WORSE: AFTER STOOL: Cocc.

Cystitis
AFTER MEDICAL INJURIES: Arn.
ATTEMPTS TO URINATE FREQUENT, MUST WAIT A LONG TIME: Arn.
ATTEMPTS TO URINATE INEFFECTUAL: Caust; Cham; Lach.
BLADDER, IRRITATION OF: Bell.
BLADDER, MUST KEEP MIND ON NECK OF, OR SHE WILL PASS URINE: Sep.
BLADDER, SENSITIVE TO JAR: Bell.
BLADDER, SENSITIVE TO PRESSURE: Bell.
CONSTANT BEARING DOWN SENSATION: Lyc.
HEAVINESS OF BLADDER: Lyc.
PAIN IN BLADDER, BURNING WHEN URINATING: Cham.
PAIN IN BLADDER, NECK OF, WHEN NOT URINATING: Cham.
PAIN IN BLADDER REGION: Apis; Caust.
RETENTION FROM COLD: Caust.
RETENTION WHEN NURSING: Apis.
URGING, CONSTANT, WHILE URINE PASSES IN DROPS: Arn.
URGING, FREQUENT: Caust.
URGING, MUST WAIT A LONG TIME: Lyc.
URINATION, AFTER LYING DOWN AND AFTER SLEEP: Lach.

URINATION, INVOLUNTARY IN SLEEP: Lyc.
URINATION, PAINFUL: Apis.
URINATION, SCANTY: Apis.
URINE, ACRID: Bell.
URINE, BLACKISH: Lach.
URINE, BLOODY: Apis; Bell.
URINE, BURNING: Bell.
URINE, BURNING ON PASSING: Lach.
URINE, CLOTTED: Bell.
URINE, COPIOUS, RED SAND IN: Lyc.
URINE, DARK BROWN: Lach.
URINE, DRIBBLING: Bell.
URINE, FOAMY: Lach.
URINE, HOT: Cham.
URINE, RED: Bell; Cham.
URINE, SUPPRESSED, ALMOST: Apis.
URINE, THICK WITH PUS: Arn.
URINE, TURBID: Cham; Lyc.
URINE, VOIDING AGONY: Apis.
URINE, WITH OFFENSIVE MUCUS: Lach.

Depression
ABSENCE OF ALL JOY: Sep.
AFRAID TO BE ALONE: Lyc.
ANXIOUS ABOUT ILLNESS: Nit Ac.
APATHETIC: China.
AVERSION TO OCCUPATION: Sep.
BEFORE PERIODS: Nat M; Nit Ac; Sep.
CANNOT BEAR EXCITEMENT: China.
CANNOT BEAR NOISE: China.
CONFUSED WITH FEELING OF WEIGHT ON HEAD: Cim.
DEPRESSED ABOUT DOMESTIC AFFAIRS: Sep.
DEPRESSED ABOUT HEALTH: Sep.
DEPRESSED WITH PREMONITION OF DEATH: Apis.
DEPRESSED WITH CONSTANT WEEPING WITHOUT CAUSE: Apis.
DESPAIR: Sep.
DESPAIR, HOPELESS: Nit Ac.
DESPAIR, OF RECOVERY: Ars.
DESPAIR, WITH FITS OF RAGE: Nit Ac.

DISTRUSTFUL: Lyc.
DREAD OF DEATH: Plat.
DREAD OF DEATH ON GOING TO BED: Ars.
DURING PREGNANCY: Nat M.
EXTREME NERVOUS IRRITABILITY: China.
FAULT FINDING: Lyc.
FULL OF RUSH AND TORMENT: Lil T.
GRIEVING: Cim.
HURRIED: Lil T.
IMPULSE TO KILL OR COMMIT SUICIDE: Merc.
INDIFFERENT: China; Lil T; Sep.
MELANCHOLY: Ars; Lyc; Phos.
MENTAL DISTURBANCE AFTER FRIGHT: Plat.
MENTAL DISTURBANCE AFTER GRIEF: Plat.
MENTAL DISTURBANCE AFTER VEXATION: Plat.
MIND, DISTURBED BY BUSINESS FAILURE: Cim.
MIND, DISTURBED BY DISAPPOINTED LOVE: Cim.
MIND, FULL OF IMPENDING EVIL: Merc.
MIND, TIRED: Lyc.
MIND, WANDERING: Nit Ac.
MIND, WEAK: Nit Ac.
MIND, WORRIED: Lyc.
MOODY: Nat M.
SENSATION OF HEAVY CLOUD: Cim.
SIGHING: Cim.
SUSPICIOUS: Cim.
TACITURN: Cim.
TROUBLED: Cim.
WEEPY: Lil T.

WORSE, IN WARM ROOM: Apis.
WORSE, AT NIGHT WITH SWEATS: Merc.

Diarrhoea
ANUS, BURNING: Cham.
ANUS, CLOTS OF BLOOD FROM: Alum.
ANUS, SORENESS: Bry.
AUTUMNAL DIARRHOEA WITH GRIPING: Ip.
DIARRHOEA AND CONSTIPATION ALTERNATING: Lach.
DURING THE DAY MOSTLY: Nat M.

AT NIGHT WITH COLIC: Sul.

STOOLS, ACRID: Bry.

STOOLS, BILIOUS: Bry.

STOOLS, BLOODY: Apis; Ip; Merc; Nat M; Nit Ac; Sec; Phos; Puls.

STOOLS, BROWNISH: China; Nat M.

STOOLS, CHALK-LIKE: Pod.

STOOLS, CHANGEABLE: Puls.

STOOLS, CHRONIC: Nat M.

STOOLS, CLAY-COLOURED: Merc.

STOOLS, COPIOUS: Phos.

STOOLS, CORROSIVE: Puls.

STOOLS, DARK: Lach: Merc.

STOOLS, DEBILITATING: Sep.

STOOLS, DRIVING OUT OF BED, MORNINGS: Sul.

STOOLS, FERMENTED: Ip.

STOOLS, FREQUENT: Calc; Cham; Pod.

STOOLS, FROTHY: China.

STOOLS, GREEN: Cham; Ip; Merc; Nat M; Nit Ac; Phos; Pod; Sec; Sil.

STOOLS, GREEN MUCUS: Sep.

STOOLS, GREENISH-YELLOW: Puls.

STOOLS, GREY: Calc.

STOOLS, GRIPING: Apis.

STOOLS, GUSHING: Pod.

STOOLS, INVOLUNTARY: China; Nat M; Sec; Sulph.

STOOLS, JELLY-LIKE: Sep.

STOOLS, LIKE DIRTY WATER: Bry.

STOOLS, LIQUID: Calc.

STOOLS, MUCO-GELATINOUS: Pod.

STOOLS, OFFENSIVE: Apis; Ars; Calc; China; Lach; Merc; Puls.

STOOLS, PAINFUL: Cham Ip.

STOOLS, PAINLESS: Apis; Ars; China; Ip; Phos; Pod; Sul.

STOOLS, PAINLESS WITH GREAT EXHAUSTION: Sil.

STOOLS, PALE: Lyc.

STOOLS, PASTY: Bry; Calc.

STOOLS, PITCH-LIKE: Merc.

STOOLS, PROFUSE: Phos.

STOOLS, PUTRID: Lyc; Nit Ac; Sec.

STOOLS, REDDISH-YELLOW: Lyc.

STOOLS, SLIMY: Merc; Nit Ac; Puls.

STOOLS, SOUR SMELLING: Calc; Merc; Pod; Sep.
STOOLS, TENACIOUS: Merc.
STOOLS, THIN: Cham; Lyc; Sec.
STOOLS, UNDIGESTED FOOD: Merc; Pod.
STOOLS, UNDIGESTED FOOD WITH MUCH THIRST DURING NIGHT: Phos.
STOOLS, WATERY: Apis; Ars; Calc; Cham; Lach; Nat M; Phos; Pod; Puls; Sul.
STOOLS, WHITE MUCUS: Puls.
STOOLS, WHITE PAPESCENT: China; Sil.
STOOLS, WHITISH: Calc.
STOOLS, YELLOW: Apis; Calc; China; Ip; Lyc; Merc; Pod.
STOOLS, YELLOW-WHITE FLUID: Nit Ac.
WITH DRY MOUTH: Nat M.
WITH FEVER: Nat M.
WITH ICY COLDNESS: Sec.
WITH MUCUS: Cham; Merc; Nit Ac.
WITH MUCUS GREEN: Ip.
WITH NAUSEA: Ip.
WITH THIRST: Nat M.
WITH URGING IN RECTUM WHEN URINATING: Alum.
WITH WEAKNESS, EXTREME: Apis.
WITH WHITE GRANULATED SEDIMENT: Bry.

Haemorrhoids
BLEEDING: Calc; Phos; Puls.
BLEEDING AFTER EVERY STOOL: Nit Ac.
BLIND: Nux V; Sul.
CHRONIC: Nit Ac.
DURING PREGNANCY: Pod.
FLOWING DARK BLOOD: Sul.
IMPENDING STOOL: Caust.
ITCHING: Alum; Caust; Graph; Lach; Nux V; Sul.
LARGE: Graph.
MOIST: Caust.
PAIN, ACHING: Calc.
PAIN, BURNING: Alum; Ars; Caust; Nux V; Sul.
PAIN, EXCORIATING: Sul.
PAIN, IN RECTUM SOME HOURS AFTER STOOL: Nux V.
PAIN, PULSATING IN ANUS: Sul.

PAIN, SMARTING: Nux V; Puls.
PAIN, SORE: Puls.
PAIN, SORE TO TOUCH: Graph.
PAIN, STICKING: Nux V.
PAIN, STINGING: Apis; Caust; Sul.
PAIN, STINGING ESPECIALLY AFTER CONFINEMENT: Apis.
PAIN, STITCHING WHILE SITTING: Ars.
PAIN, STITCHING WHILE WALKING: Ars; Caust.
PAIN, TAKING WIDE STEP: Graph.
PAINFUL: Calc; Nux V; Puls; Sil.
PAINFUL WHEN TOUCHED: Caust; Nit Ac.
PAINFUL WHEN WALKING: Calc; Caust.
PENDULOUS: Nit Ac.
PROTRUDING: Calc; Lach; Puls.
PROTRUDING DURING STOOL: Sil.
PROTRUDING LIKE COALS OF FIRE: Ars.
SLIMY: Nit Ac.
STRANGULATED: Lach.
SWOLLEN: Caust.
SWOLLEN ANUS: Sul.

BETTER, AFTER NIGHT'S REST: Alum.
BETTER, HEAT (BURNING PAINS): Ars.
BETTER, SITTING: Calc.

WORSE, EVENINGS: Alum.
WORSE, WARM WEATHER: Nit Ac.

Headaches
BAND SENSATION: Nit Ac.
BILIOUS: Sep; Sil; Sul.
BLINDING: Nat M.
CATARRHAL: Merc.
CHRONIC: Lach; Nat M; Phos; Sil.
CONGESTIVE: Ars; Bell; China; Gels; Lach; Nux V; Phos.
FROM OVERWORK: Puls.
FROM WASHING HAIR: Bell.
HEAVINESS OF HEAD: Acon; Sul.
NERVOUS: Sep.
NEURALGIC: Ars; Gels; Puls; Sep; Sul.
NUMBNESS OF HEAD: Calc.

PAIN, ACHING: Arn.
PAIN, BURNING: Acon; Apis; Arn.
PAIN, BURSTING: Bell; Bry; China; Cocc.
PAIN, CRUSHING: Bry.
PAIN, CUTTING: Arn; Bell.
PAIN, DARTING: Phos.
PAIN, HAMMERING: Gels.
PAIN, PRESSING: Lyc; Pod; Sul.
PAIN, SHOOTING: Arn; Bell; Phos.
PAIN, SPLITTING: Bry.
PAIN, STABBING: Bell.
PAIN, STINGING: Apis.
PAIN, STITCHING: Nux V; Puls.
PAIN, TEARING: Acon; Merc; Phos.
PAIN, THROBBING: Bell; China; Lach; Lyc; Nat M; Phos.
PAIN, VIOLENT: Acon; Bell; Gels; Phos; Sep.
PAIN, WANDERING: Puls.
PAIN, FOREHEAD, FULLNESS: Acon.
PAIN, FOREHEAD, STITCHING: China.
PAIN, FOREHEAD, TEARING: Calc.
PAIN, FRONTAL: Puls.
PAIN, OCCIPUT, FROM TO WHOLE OF HEAD: China.
PAIN, OCCIPUT, OPENING AND SHUTTING: Cocc.
PAIN, OCCIPUT, SHARP: Apis.
PAIN, OCCIPUT, TEARING: Lyc.
PAIN, OCCIPUT, VERY BAD: Ars.
PAIN, OCCIPUT, WITH VOMITING AND NAUSEA: Sep.
PAIN, TEMPLES AS IF SCREWED TOGETHER: Lyc.
PAIN, TEMPLES STITCHING: China.
PAIN, VERTEX BURNING: Sul.
PAIN, VERTEX, PRESSURE ON: Lach; Lyc; Puls.
PAIN, VERTEX PULSATING: Cocc.
PERIODIC: Ars; Phos; Sep.
WITH NAUSEA: Ars.
WITH VOMITING: Ars.

BETTER, APPLIED HEAT: Sep; Sil.
BETTER, BATHING IN COLD WATER: Ars.
BETTER, COPIOUS URINATION: Gels.
BETTER, FRESH AIR: Lyc.

BETTER, HARD EXERCISE: Sep.
BETTER, INDOORS: Cocc.
BETTER, LYING: Sep.
BETTER, PRESSURE: Bell; Sil.
BETTER, PRESSURE, HARD: China.
BETTER, REST: Cocc.
BETTER, WARMTH: Nux V.
BETTER, WRAPPING UP HEAD: Nux V; Sil.

WORSE, 4–8 pm: Lyc.
WORSE, DRAUGHT: China.
WORSE, DRINKING: Cocc; Sul.
WORSE, EATING: Cocc; Nux V; Sul.
WORSE, HEAT: Phos.
WORSE, JAR: Bell; SEP.
WORSE, LIGHT: Bell; Phos; Sep.
WORSE, LYING DOWN: Bell.
WORSE, MORNING ON WAKING: Nat M; Nux V; Pod.
WORSE, MOTION: Bell; Bry; Sul.
WORSE, NOISE: Bell; Phos.
WORSE, SLEEPING: Lach.
WORSE, SMELL OF FOOD: Cocc.
WORSE, STOOPING: Bell; Sep.

Leucorrhoea
ACRID: Ars; Bor; Cham; Graph; Kreos; Lyc; Merc; Nat M; Nit Ac; Phos; Puls; Sep; Sil.
AFTER PERIODS: Nit Ac.
ALBUMINOUS: Nat M; Sep.
BLOODY: China; Merc; Nit Ac; Sep.
BROWN: Lil T; Nit Ac; Sec.
BURNING: Alum; Bor; Calc; Kreos; Lyc; Puls; Sep; Sul.
COPIOUS: Acon; Calc; Graph; Sep; Sil.
CORRODING: Ars.
CREAM-LIKE: Puls.
EXCORIATING: Ars; Bor; Cham; Graph; Kreos; Lyc; Merc; Nit Ac; Phos; Puls; Sep; Sil; Sul.
GREENISH: Merc; Nat M; Sep.
GUSHING: Calc; Cocc; Lyc; Sep; Sil.
GUSHING, AFTER MENSES: Graph.

INSTEAD OF PERIODS: Phos.
MILKY: Calc; Sep; Sil.
MUCUS: Caul.
OFFENSIVE: Nit Ac; Nux V; Sep.
OFFENSIVE IN PREGNANCY: Sep.
PROFUSE: Alum; Ars; Caul; Caust; Phos.
PURULENT: Cocc.
PUTRID IN PREGNANCY: Kreos.
ROPY: Alum; Nit Ac; Sab.
STRINGY: Nit Ac; Sab.
TENACIOUS: Acon; Nit Ac; Sab.
THICK: Ars; Calc.
THIN: Nit Ac.
TRANSPARENT: Nat M; Sep.
WATERY: Graph; Nat M; Nit Ac.
WHITE: Graph; Nat M; Sep.
WITH, ITCHING: Kreos; Nit Ac; Sep.
WITH, ITCHING AND BURNING: Calc.
WITH, LABOUR-LIKE PAINS: Kali C.
WITH, RAWNESS IN PARTS: Merc.
WITH, SMARTING: Phos.
WITH, WEAKNESS: Cocc; Graph.
YELLOWISH: Acon; Cham; Kreos; Sep; Sul.
YELLOWISH: WITH BACKACHE: Kali C.

BETTER, WASHING IN COLD WATER: Alum.

WORSE, DAYTIME: Alum.
WORSE, MORNING: Sep.
WORSE, NIGHT: Caust; Merc.
WORSE, WALKING: Nit Ac.

Menopause
WITH ANXIETY: Sep.
WITH BILIOUSNESS: Kali C.
WITH BLEEDING BETWEEN PERIODS: Calc.
WITH FAINTING: Lach; Nux M; Sep; Sul.
WITH FLOODING: Cim; Nit Ac; Sep.
WITH FLOODING BETWEEN PERIOD TIME: Calc; Lach.
WITH FLUSHES OF HEAT: Acon; Bor; Bell; Cim; Kali C; Lach; Nux V; Phos; Sep; Sul.

WITH FLUSHES OF HEAT FOLLOWED BY CHILLINESS: Caust.
WITH FLUSHES OF HEAT TRAVELLING UPWARDS: Calc.
WITH HEADACHE: Cim; Lach; Sep.
WITH HEAT OF FACE: Graph.
WITH LOSS OF APPETITE: Kali C.
WITH MENTAL DEPRESSION: Cim; Lach.
WITH NOSE BLEED: Graph.
WITH RUSH OF BLOOD TO HEAD: Graph.
WITH TASTE OF BILE IN MOUTH ON WAKING: Kali C.
WITH WEAKNESS: Lach.

Menses (Periods)
ABSENT: Apis; Con; Graph; Kali C; Lyc; Phos; Puls; Sab; Sil.
CEASE WHEN LYING: Lil T.
DAYTIME ONLY: Puls.
DEBILITY BETWEEN PERIODS: Cim.
DIMINISHED: Acon.
DISCHARGE ACRID: Kali C; Lach; Sil; Sul.
DISCHARGE BLACK: Lach; Puls; Sul.
DISCHARGE BROWN: Bry.
DISCHARGE CHANGEABLE IN APPEARANCE: Puls.
DISCHARGE CLOTTED: Calc; Caust; Cham; Ip; Lach; Plat; Puls; Sab.
DISCHARGE COAGULATED: Cim.
DISCHARGE COPIOUS: Bell; Calc; China; Cocc; Ip; Nux V; Nux M; Nat M; Phos; Plat; Sab.
DISCHARGE COPIOUS WHEN STANDING: Cocc.
DISCHARGE COPIOUS WHEN WALKING: Cocc.
DISCHARGE COPIOUS WITH FAINTNESS: Ip.
DISCHARGE DARK: Bell; Cham; Cim; Nux M; Nux V; Plat; Puls; Sec.
DISCHARGE DARK CLOTS: China.
DISCHARGE LIKE MUDDY WATER: Nit Ac.
DISCHARGE MAKING PARTS SORE: Sul.
DISCHARGE MEMBRANOUS: Cham.
DISCHARGE OFFENSIVE: Ars; Bry; Bell; Cim; Kreos; Sab.
DISCHARGE PALE: Alum; Ars; Graph; Kali C; Nat M.
DISCHARGE PROFUSE: Ars; Bor; Bry; Caul; Caust; Cim; Lyc; Nit Ac; Sep.
DISCHARGE RED, BRIGHT: Bell; Ip; Phos.

DISCHARGE THICK: Nux M; Puls; Sul.
DISCHARGE THIN: Ars; Nat M.
DISCHARGE WHITE: Ars.
DISCHARGE WITH BAD ODOUR: Caust.
DURATION SHORT: Lach; Puls; Sul
EARLY, TOO: Alum; Ars; Bell; Bor; Bry; Caul; Caust; Cocc; Ip; Nux V; Sab; Sep.
EXCESSIVE: Apis.
EXHAUSTION, FOLLOWED BY GREAT: Alum.
FAINTNESS: Apis.
FIRST PERIOD DIFFICULT: Kali C.
FIRST PERIOD IN GIRLS, DELAYED: Graph, Kali C; Nat M; Puls.
FREQUENT: Calc; Cham; Ip; Kali C; Nat M; Nux M; Nux V; Phos; Plat; Sab.
HEADACHE, OFTEN PRECEDED BY: Alum.
HEARING DIFFICULT DURING: Kreos.
INTERMITS: Kreos.
INTERMITTENT: Puls.
IRREGULAR: Cim; Nat M; Nux M; Nux V; Sec.
ITCHING BEFORE: Graph.
LATE: Acon; Con; Graph; Lyc; Nat M; Nux M; Puls; Sep; Sil; Sul.
LONGER LASTING: Kali C.
MENTAL TROUBLES ASSOCIATED WITH SUPPRESSED PERIODS: Plat.
PAIN, BEARING DOWN: Sep.
PAIN, BEFORE PERIOD (IMMEDIATELY): Cim.
PAIN, COLIC WITH COLDNESS: Sep.
PAIN, CRAMPING: Cocc; Graph.
PAIN, CUTTING: Cocc.
PAIN, LABOUR-LIKE: Cim.
PAIN, SHARP: Cim.
PAINFUL: Apis; Ars; Bell; Caul; Cham; Gels; Kali C.
PAINFUL ON GETTING FEET WET: Puls.
PROLONGED: Kali C; Kreos; Lach; Nat M; Nit Ac; Nux M; Phos; Puls; Sep; Sul.
PROTRACTED: Acon; Calc; Kreos; Lyc; Nat M; Nux V; Plat; Puls; Sab.
RESTLESSNESS: Apis.
SCANTY: Alum; Ars; Con; Gels; Graph; Kali C.
STOPS AT NIGHT: Caust.

SUPPRESSED: Bell; Bry; Con; Graph; Lach; Lyc; Nat M; Pod; Puls; Sil.
SUPPRESSED FROM FRIGHT: Acon.
UNEASINESS: Apis.
WEAK DURING PERIODS: Cocc.
WITH COLIC: Bor.
WITH NAUSEA: Bor.

BETTER, FOR PERIODS: Nux M.
BETTER, WHEN FLOW STARTS: Lach.

WORSE, AFTER PERIODS: Bor; Kreos.
WORSE, DURING PERIODS: Cim; Graph; Nux V.

Metrorrhagia (Bleeding from Uterus between periods)
AFTER EXERTION: Calc.
AFTER LABOUR: Ip; Sab.
AFTER SEXUAL INTERCOURSE: Kreos.
AT MENOPAUSE: Calc; Lach; Sep; Sul.
BETWEEN PERIODS: Calc.
BETWEEN PERIODS AFTER CHILDBIRTH: Nit Ac.
BLACK: Plat.
BRIGHT RED: Ip.
BRIGHT RED FROM FIBROIDS: Phos.
COAGULATED WITH CLOTS: Bell; Cham.
CONTINUOUS OOZING OF WATERY BLOOD UNTIL NEXT PERIOD: Sec.
DARK BLOOD: China.
DURING LABOUR: Sab.
DURING LABOUR, PROFUSE: Ip.
FLUID: Lach.
FLUID, GUSHING: Phos.
FROM ANGER: Cham.
GUSHING: Ip.
INTERMITTENT: Phos.
PAROXYSMS: Sab.
PROFUSE: Bell; Calc; Phos.
SUDDEN: Bell.
WHEN PHYSICALLY ACTIVE: Bell; Ip; Phos; Sab.

Miscarriage
AROUND 2nd MONTH: Apis, Kali C.
AROUND 3rd MONTH: Merc.
DURING EARLY MONTHS: Apis.
FLOW CEASES THEN RETURNS IN FORCE, THEN CEASES
AND SO ON: Puls.
FROM FRIGHT: Gels.
FROM INJURIES: Arn.
HABITUAL FROM UTERUS DEBILITY: Caul.
TENDENCY TO: Calc; Cim; Kali C; Nux M; Sul.
TENDENCY TO, ESPECIALLY IN 3rd MONTH: Merc; Sab.
TENDENCY TO, ESPECIALLY AROUND 5th–7th MONTHS: Sep.
THREATENED ABOUT 3rd MONTH: Sec.
THREATENED FROM FRIGHT: Acon; Puls.
WITH ANXIETY: Acon.
WITH DRY SKIN: Acon.
WITH FEAR: Acon.
WITH FEVER: Acon.
WITH RESTLESSNESS: Acon.
WITH THIRST: Acon.
Belladonna is useful if other symptoms agree.

Ovaries
CONGESTED: Acon; Apis.
ENLARGED: Apis; Bell; Con; Lyc.
HEAVY, FEELS: China.
INFLAMMATION: Apis; Bell; Con; Lyc; Merc; Phos; Pod.
INFLAMMATION AFTER MISCARRIAGE: Sab.
INFLAMMATION WITH STERILITY: Plat.
PAIN AFTER LABOUR: Lach.
PAIN, BEARING DOWN WHILST STANDING: Lil T.
PAIN, BORING: Lyc.
PAIN, BURNING: Ars; Lach.
PAIN, BURNING AFTER INTERCOURSE: Apis.
PAIN, DRAWING: Ars.
PAIN, LANCINATING: Apis; Lil T.
PAIN, PRESSING: Lach.
PAIN, SHARP: Lil T.
PAIN, SHARP WHILE NURSING: Sil.
PAIN, SORE: Bry; Lach; Lil T.

PAIN, SORE IN RIGHT OVARY: Bell; Lyc; Pod.
PAIN, SORE IN RIGHT OVARY, WORSE MOTION: Bell.
PAIN, STINGING: Apis; Lil T; Merc.
PAIN, STITCHING: Ars; Bry; Graph; Lach.
PAIN, TENDER: Lach; Lil T.

WORSE, MOTION: Ars.
WORSE, LEFT OVARY: Lach.

Pregnancy

AFTER LABOUR WHEN LONG AND SLOW: Caust.
AFTER PAINS INTENSE: Sab.
AFTER PAINS LAST TOO LONG: Acon.
AFTER PAINS PAINFUL, TOO: Acon.
AFTER PAINS VIOLENT: Arn.
AFTER PAINS WITH GREAT SENSITIVENESS: Cim.
AFTER PAINS WITH NAUSEA: Cim.
AFTER PAINS VOMITING: Cim.
AFTER PREGNANCY, FOR RELIEF AND COMFORT: Arn.
AFTER PREGNANCY TO AVOID SEPSIS: Arn.
AVERSION TO COMPANY DURING: Lach.
CONFUSION OF MIND FROM MENTAL EXERTION: Nux M.
CONTRACTIONS INSUFFICIENT: Acon.
DURING, ANXIETY: Ars.
DURING, FEAR OF DEATH: Acon.
DURING LABOUR NO EXPULSION THOUGH EVERYTHING
RELAXED: Sec.
RESTLESS: Acon; Ars.
FALSE LABOUR-LIKE PAINS: Cim; Gels.
FREQUENT URGING TO STOOL: Nux V.
FREQUENT URINATION: Nux V.
LABOUR PAINS CEASING: Cim.
LABOUR PAINS RAPID: Acon.
LABOUR PAINS SEVERE: Cim.
LABOUR PAINS SHARP: Acon.
LABOUR PAINS SPASMODIC: Cim; Gels.
LABOUR PAINS TEDIOUS: Cim.
LABOUR PAINS VIOLENT: Acon.
LABOUR PAINS WEAK: Cim; Gels.
MORNING SICKNESS WITH MUCH NAUSEA: Ip.

MORNING SICKNESS WITH PROFUSE SALIVA: Merc.
NAUSEA: Cim.
OVER-STRETCHED BLADDER: Caust.
PAINS, BRUISED, AFTER LABOUR: Arn.
PAINS, GRIPING: Gels.
PAINS, LABOUR-LIKE: Gels.
SICKNESS WITH INTENSE THIRST FOR LONG COLD DRINKS:
Phos.
VOMITING: Ars; Kreos; Nux V.
VOMITING AND SICKNESS: Sul.
VOMITING 5–10 MINUTES AFTER COLD DRINK: Phos.
VOMITING WITH INTENSE SLEEPINESS: Nux M.
VOMITING WITH IRRITABILITY: Nux V.
WITH DEPRESSION: Nat M.
WITH INVOLUNTARY URINATION: Ars; Nat M; Sep.
WITH VERTIGO: Nat M.

Pre-Menstrual Tension
DEPRESSION: Calc; Caust; Cim; Cocc; Con; Lyc; Nat M; Nit Ac;
Phos; Puls; Sep.
GIDDY FEELINGS: Calc; Nux V.
HEADACHE: Bry; Cim; Cocc; Gels; Graph; Kreos; Lach; Nat M;
Nux V; Puls; Sep; Sul.
HYSTERIA: Caul; Nux V; Plat; Puls.
IRRITABLE: Cham; Cocc; Kreos; Lil T; Lyc; Nux V.
NAUSEA, INTENSE, AND MORNING SICKNESS, WORSE
ODOURS: Sep.
NERVOUS: Acon; Cham; Cim; Kreos; Lach; Nit Ac; Puls.
NERVOUS RESTLESSNESS: Sep.
STOMACH DISTURBANCE: Bry; Kali C; Lach; Lyc; Nux V; Puls;
Sep; Sul.
WEAKNESS: Alum; Cocc; Graph; Puls.
WEEPY: Phos.

Sexual Desire
AVERSION TO: Caust; Graph; Nat M; Sep.
DIMINISHED: Caust.
ENJOYMENT MISSING: Caust; Sep.
INCREASED: Calc; Con; Lach; Nux V; Phos; Plat; Puls; Sab.
INTERCOURSE PAINFUL: Lyc.
INTERCOURSE PAINFUL FROM DRYNESS: Nat M.

Sleeplessness
AFRAID TO GO TO SLEEP: Lach.
AFTER ABUSE OF ALCHOHOL: Nux V.
AFTER ABUSE OF COFFEE: Nux V.
AFTER ABUSE OF TOBACCO: Nux V.
AFTER ABUSE OF WINE: Nux V.
AFTER CHILL: Acon.
AFTER EATING TOO MUCH: Puls.
AFTER EXCITEMENT AT THEATRE: Phos.
AFTER EXERTION AND PHYSICAL STRAIN: Arn.
AFTER FRIGHT: Acon.
AFTER MENTAL STRAIN: Nux V.
AFTER SHOCK: Acon.
AWAKE UNTIL AROUND 3 am: Merc.
BED FEELS TOO HARD: Arn.
DROWSY BY DAY, WAKEFUL AT NIGHT: Sul.
DURING PREGNANCY: Cim.
EXHAUSTED BUT CANNOT SLEEP: Cocc.
FIXED IDEA PREVENTS SLEEP BEFORE MIDNIGHT: Puls.
FROM ACTIVE MIND: Bry; Calc.
FROM ANXIETY: Cocc; Lach; Merc.
FROM ANXIETY DRIVING HER OUT OF BED: Ars.
FROM DELUSIONS: Bry.
FROM EXCITEMENT: Acon.
FROM FLOW OF THOUGHTS: Sul.
FROM GREAT FEAR: Acon; Puls.
FROM GRIEF: Cocc.
FROM ITCHING: Merc.
FROM LONG NURSING: Cocc.
FROM NIGHT SWEATS: Merc.
FROM SEEING FRIGHTFUL FACES: Merc.
FROM SOLES OF FEET BURNING, PUTS THEM OUT OF BED:
Sul.
FROM THOUGHTS RUSHING INTO MIND: Sep.
FROM TOO MUCH STUDY AT NIGHT: Nux V.
FROM VEXATION: Cocc.
FROM VIOLENT PAIN: Cham.
PART LAID ON SORE: Arn.
PROLONGED LOSS OF SLEEP: Cocc.
RESTLESS: Acon; Ars; Bry; Cham; Sep.

RESTLESS WITH FRIGHTFUL DREAMS: Bell.
SLEEP, CANNOT IN SPITE OF FEELING SLEEPY: Bell.
SLEEPLESSNESS BEFORE MIDNIGHT: Bry; Phos.
SLEEPS INTO AGGRAVATION: Lach.
SLEEPY BUT CANNOT GET TO SLEEP: Cham.
SLEEPY DURING DAY, RESTLESS AT NIGHT: Phos.
SOUND SLEEP WHEN TIME TO WAKE UP: Puls.
TIRED ON WAKING: Nux V.
TOO TIRED TO SLEEP: Arn.
TOSSING ABOUT: Acon; Arn; Sul.
UNEASY AFTER MIDNIGHT: Ars.
UNEASY BEFORE MIDNIGHT: Bell.
WAKENED BY VIVID DREAMS: Phos.
WAKENS AFTER FRIGHT: Lach.
WAKENS AND CANNOT SLEEP AGAIN: Lach.
WAKENS 2 am AND CANNOT SLEEP AFTERWARDS: Kali C.
WAKENS AROUND 3 am: Sep.
WAKENS 3–4 am AND THEN SLEEP DIFFICULT: Nux V.
WAKENS 3, 4 or 5 am: Sul.
WAKENS FREQUENTLY: Merc.
WAKENS FREQUENTLY WITHOUT CAUSE: Sep.
WEEPS BECAUSE SHE CANNOT SLEEP: Puls.
WIDE AWAKE AT BEDTIME: Cham.
WITH MOANING: Ars.

BETTER, SLEEP LATE MORNING: Sul.

WORSE, BEDCLOTHES TOUCHING THROAT: Lach.
WORSE, WARMTH OF BED: Sul.
WORSE, MORNING SLEEP: Nux V.

Sterility
STERILITY: Bor; Nat M; Sep.

Subinvolution
Failure of the recently pregnant uterus to return to normal size
within the usual time; about six weeks after delivery: Bell; Calc;
Caul; Cim; Puls; Sab; Sep; Sul.

Uterus
CONGESTION: Sep.
CONGESTION AFTER PERIODS: Lach.
CONGESTION BEFORE PERIODS: Bell.
CONGESTION DURING PERIODS: Bell.
CONTRACTIONS SPASMODIC: Caul.
DISPLACEMENT: Bell; Calc; Lach; Nat M; Nit Ac; Sep.
ENLARGEMENT: Con; Sep.
FIBROIDS: Calc; Phos.
HAEMORRHAGE FROM: Nit Ac.
HAEMORRHAGE BRIGHT, WITH NAUSEA: Ip.
HAEMORRHAGE GUSHING, WITH NAUSEA: Ip.
HAEMORRHAGE PROFUSE, WITH NAUSEA: Ip.
HEAVINESS: Sep.
HEAVINESS WITH LABOUR PAINS: Cham.
INERTIA DURING LABOUR: Caust.
INFLAMMATION: Apis; Bell; Lach; Lyc; Puls.
INFLAMMATION AFTER MISCARRIAGE: Sab.
LABOUR PAINS CEASING: Kali C; Puls.
LABOUR PAINS DISTRESSING: Cham; Kali C.
LABOUR PAINS EXCESSIVE: Cham.
LABOUR PAINS AND FAINTNESS: Nux V.
LABOUR PAINS FALSE: Bell; Calc; Caul; Puls.
LABOUR PAINS INEFFECTUAL: Puls.
LABOUR PAINS IRREGULAR: Caul.
LABOUR PAINS SHORT: Caul.
LABOUR PAINS SPASMODIC: Caul; Caust; Cham.
LABOUR PAINS AND URGING TO STOOL: Nux V.
LABOUR PAINS WEAK: Kali C; Nat M; Puls.
LABOUR-LIKE PAINS: Cham; Kali C; Puls; Sep.
PAIN – AFTER PAINS: Cham, Kali C; Puls; Sab.
PAIN – AFTER PAINS SPASMODIC: Caul.
PAIN – AFTER PAINS WHEN CHILD IS NURSED: Sil.
PAIN BEARING DOWN: Bell; Cham; Cim; Kreos; Lil T; Nat M; Plat; Puls; Sab.
PAIN BEARING DOWN, BETTER CROSSING LEGS: Lil T; Sep.
PAIN BEARING DOWN, DURING PERIOD: Lil T; Sep.
PAIN BEARING DOWN, NIGHT IN BED: Sul.
PAIN BEARING DOWN, WITH URGING TO STOOL: Nux V.
PAIN, BETTER FLOW: Lach.

PAIN, BITING: Kreos.
PAIN, BURNING: Kreos; Nit Ac.
PAIN, CONSTRICTIVE: Bell.
PAIN, CRAMPING: Sab.
PAIN, CRAMPING AFTER ANGER: Cham.
PAIN, CRAMPING BEFORE MENSES: Caul; Cham; Graph.
PAIN, CRAMPING COMPELLING DOUBLING UP: Nux V.
PAIN, CRAMPING DURING MENSES: Cham; Nux V.
PAIN, CUTTING: Cocc; Puls.
PAIN, DRAWING: Bell.
PAIN, EXCESSIVE: Sep.
PAIN, FROM NAVEL TO UTERUS: Ip.
PAIN, GRIPING: Bell; Cham; Kali C; Puls; Sep.
PAIN, PAROXYSMAL: Bell; Cham; Puls; Sab.
PAIN, PERIODS, BEFORE: Calc; Kali C; Puls.
PAIN, PERIODS, DURING: Calc, Nux V; Puls.
PAIN, PINCHING: Bell.
PAIN, PRESSING: Bell.
PAIN, SORE: Bry; Bell; Kreos; Lach; Plat.
PAIN, SORE BEFORE PERIODS: Sep.
PAIN, SORE DURING INTERCOURSE: Puls.
PAIN, SORE WORSE MOTION: Bell; Bry.
PAIN, SORE WORSE WALKING: Bry.
PAIN, STITCHING: Bell; Cim; Sep.
PAIN, TENDER: Cim; Lach; Plat.
PAIN, TENDER BEFORE PERIODS: Sep.
PAIN, WANDERING: Puls.
PAIN, WHILE NURSING: Sil.
POLYPUS: Ars; Bell; Calc; Con; Lyc; Phos; Plat; Sep; Sil.
PROLAPSE: Lil T; Nat M; Nux V; Plat; Puls.
PROLAPSE DURING PERIODS: Sep.
PROLAPSE FROM OVERLIFTING DURING PREGNANCY: Pod.
PROLAPSE FROM OVER STRAINING DURING PREGNANCY: Pod.
PROLAPSE SUDDEN WITH INFLAMMATION: Acon.
RETROVERTED: Caul.
SENSATION OF CONGESTION: Caul.

Vagina
DISCHARGES CLEAR: Alum.

DISCHARGES CLEAR WITH BURNING: Alum.
DISCHARGES CLEAR WITH BURNING AND ITCHING: Alum.
DRY: Acon; Lyc; Nat M; Sep.
HOT: Acon.
INFLAMMATION OF: Acon; Merc; Nit Ac; Sep; Sul.
IRRITABLE: Caul.
ITCHING: Bor; Calc; Caust; Con; Graph; Kali C; Kreos; Lil T; Lyc; Nat M; Sil; Sul.
ITCHING FROM LEUCORRHOEA AFTER PREGNANCY: Sep.
ITCHING, VIOLENT, WORSE URINATING: Kreos.
PAIN AFTER INTERCOURSE: Sep.
PAIN, BURNING: Lyc; Nit Ac; Sul.
PAIN, INTENSE: Caul.
PAIN, SORENESS: Bor; Kreos.
PAIN, SPASMODIC: Caul.
PAIN, STITCHING: Nit Ac.
PAIN, TENDER: Kreos.
PAIN, THROBBING, LEFT SIDE: Alum.
POLYPUS: Calc; Puls.
PROLAPSE: Sep.
SENSITIVE: Acon; Plat; Sil.
ULCERATION: Caul.

Varicose Ulcers
BLUISH, PURPLISH: Lach.
BURNING: Ars; Sil.
BURNING, WORSE AT NIGHT: Lyc; Nit Ac; Puls.
DEEP: Ars; Calc.
DURING PREGNANCY: Arn.
FOOT, IN: Graph; Puls.
LEGS, IN: Graph, Kali C; Lach; Puls.
PAINFUL: Ars; Lach; Puls.
TOES IN, ORIGINATING IN BLISTERS: Graph.

WORSE, NIGHT: Sil.
WORSE, WARMTH: Merc; Puls.

Varicose Veins
DURING PREGNANCY: Arn; Ars; Graph.
INFLAMED: Calc.
LEGS, ESPECIALLY IN: Nat M.

LOWER LIMBS, ESPECIALLY IN: Kreos.
PAINFUL: Lyc; Puls.
STINGING DURING PREGNANCY: Puls.
WITH ULCERATION: Lach.

Vulva
INFLAMMATION: Calc.
ITCHING: Alum; Bor; Calc; Sil.
ITCHING AND BURNING: Kali C.
ITCHING, CORROSIVE: Kreos.
PAIN, BEARING DOWN: Lil T.
PAIN, SORE: Alum; Calc; Kreos.
PAIN, WORSE STANDING: Sep.
PAIN, WORSE URGING TO URINATE: Sep.
SENSITIVE: Sil.
SWELLING: Calc.

CONTRACEPTIVES

Contraceptives are in general use these days and most women with whom I have contact use one of them; there is a choice.

Everybody has a right to choose for themselves whether they use contraceptives or not but I would like to say something about the Pill.

Many people have stopped using it on my advice and anybody coming to me as a patient who is using the Pill goes away knowing that I disapprove very strongly.

Within the last two weeks a report has appeared in the press of the death of a girl of 17 from using the Pill, and another report by a doctor who has been working on the Pill for 25 years saying it is not safe. This woman doctor admits that she, like many others, welcomed the discovery of the Pill 25 years ago. But ten years later she realized that through those years much ill-health in women was Pill induced.

Research has found that alterations in developing bone marrow increase the danger of infection and allergy, and there is a greater risk of thrombosis, strokes, haemorrhages and heart attacks.

Of course this will be denied and contradicted by other doctors and drug manufacturers but, if any drug is taken over a long period side effects often become evident because drugs are foreign to the human body, they are artificial and work against all the laws of nature, obstructing the work of the built-in natural healing forces which are trying all the time to keep every human being healthy.

Throughout the years many women have come for help in varying states, being disturbed not only physically but feeling depressed and wretched mentally and by giving up the Pill they have blossomed into healthy, happy people.

Do think very seriously if you are taking the Pill. There are other contraceptives to choose from.

THE IMPORTANCE OF FOOD

A good healthy food programme is important. 'Whole food is one of the avenues to health and vitality', says Boris Chaitow in his excellent book *My Healing Secrets*. He is an expert in nutrition and a man who carries out everything that he recommends.

So let us examine whole foods:

Bread is something that most of us consume and should be made from 100 per cent wholemeal flour. Nothing has been extracted from this flour and so it contains all the bran (roughage) and wheatgerm. If the wheat has been grown organically then the bread is even more nutritious;

100 per cent self-raising wholemeal flour is obtainable at most Health Food Stores and this should be used for scones, cakes (yes, even sponge cakes!), biscuits and flans, both sweet and savoury. All white flour products should be avoided;

Sugar should be cut to a minimum. When molasses is taken from the sugar cane it is a wholesome product, containing vitamins and minerals needed for health, but most of it is processed until it arrives on the shop shelves in packets – pristine white, having been bleached as well. It sweetens, certainly, but to quote Boris Chaitow again 'In all cases of nervous instability, tendency to sensitivity, nervous tension, being highly strung, emotional, variable moods and energy, subject to bouts of depression or any combinations or variations of these destructive effects, are adversely exaggerated by the use of sugar or sugar products'.

There is a little raw brown sugar on the market which is better than most but honey is the best alternative although this should not be consumed in large quantities;

Some uncooked food should be taken every day, a good salad containing some of the following ingredients – lettuce, chinese leaves, watercress, mustard and cress, chicory, grated raw white cabbage, grated raw carrots and raw beetroot, cucumber, radishes, mushrooms, chopped raw cauliflower, onions, with lemon and oil dressing. Some sunflower seeds and nuts may be added, or some cheese, preferably cottage cheese, or a jacket potato. A chopped apple or some raisins give a different flavour – there can be a great variety in salads.

A savoury dish or a little chicken, fish, meat or an egg dish should be taken at the second meal with cooked vegetables. If a sweet is needed fresh fruit is best;

Tea and coffee should be limited and milk cut to the minimum as this is mucus forming, this applies to cheese also. Natural fruit juices (unsweetened) are excellent;

The following should be avoided: refined and processed foods, foods containing additives, artificial colouring and preservatives; sweets, chocolate, pies, pasties, pickles;

The following should be eaten and drunk in moderation: meat, cheese, fats, alcohol, tea and coffee.

For those interested in further study of nutrition and health I suggest that *My Healing Secrets* by Boris Chaitow (published by Health Science Press) is excellent.

MIND USE AND HEALTH

I cannot finish this book without saying something about our thoughts in connection with our health.

All thought, whether positive or negative, affects our health.

The mind is not in a separate compartment in the body, we are our minds and our physical bodies are reflections of the mind.

In other words if we are happy and thinking positively – I prefer to say 'creatively' – our physical bodies are being healed, and if we think about this for a moment, we know that when we are happy and contented we feel good! On the other hand if we are angry, irritable, discontented or resentful – negative states – then we feel wretched and depressed, but at the same time poisons are being released into the body, literally reaching every cell, and so the level of health is lowered, and if we are continually in this negative state we become ill.

We are, in fact, discovering that every one of our thoughts is important.

There is no doubt that negative thoughts come so much more easily, they seem more comfortable than those that are creative. How often do you think to yourself or hear other people say 'I ought not to do that', 'I'm sure I'm going to have a cold', 'I shouldn't eat that it will upset me', 'I'm never well in the spring'! Negative thoughts are endless and often we don't even appreciate that they are negative, we take them all for granted.

To think creatively is even more important when we are ill. And the key to this is daily meditation.

If we sit quietly, completely relaxing and letting go of all tensions and strains for a few minutes each day and think of something creative – Light, Love, Peace or Joy for instance – and visualize ourselves with Light flowing towards and into us, we set the healing forces in motion. This quiet time, or meditation, is so important because it is the only time we choose our thoughts, and so we can choose to think creatively.

Our daily quiet period will not only help us to feel better but it will help us to cope with our daily life. We shall enjoy each day, we shall be able to achieve more, we shall feel more peaceful.

This is no fairy tale, it is reality. I have introduced 'Mind-use' to many patients who have been amazed at the results. Not only do they feel much better in health but they don't get so worried about things and they become far less stressed and strained.

Stresses and tensions are so common these days – they are the cause of many complaints from which women suffer and there is no doubt that a great deal of ill-health could be avoided if we 'let go' and begin to think creatively.

To change our thought processes makes life very exciting and improves our health.

For more information I recommend *The A.B.C. of Health and Healing* by Jack Burton, MA, published by and obtainable from The Book Dept, Maillard House Trust, Manor House, Coffinswell, Devon TQ12 4SW.